PUBLISHED BY ALFRED A. KNOPF CANADA

www.penguinrandomhouse.ca

Knopf Canada and colophon are registered trademarks.

Library and Archives Canada Cataloguing in Publication

Title: An alphabet for Joanna : a portrait of my mother in 26 fragments / Damian Rogers.
Names: Rogers, Damian, author.
Identifiers: Canadiana (print) 20189045787 | Canadiana (ebook) 20189045795 |
ISBN 9780735273030 (hardcover) | ISBN 9780735273054 (EPUB)
Subjects: LCSH: Rogers, Damian. | LCSH: Rogers, Damian—Family. | LCSH:
Mothers and daughters. | LCSH: Children of mentally ill mothers—Canada—
Biography. | LCSH: Mentally ill mothers—Canada—Biography. | CSH: Poets,
Canadian (English)—Biography.
Classification: LCC PS8635 O425 Z46 2020 | DDC C811/.6—dc23

Text design: Kate Sinclair
Jacket art and design: Kate Sinclair

Printed and bound in Canada

10 9 8 7 6 5 4 3 2 1

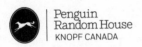

Penguin
Random House
KNOPF CANADA

AN
ALPHABET
FOR
JOANNA

A PORTRAIT OF MY MOTHER
IN 26 FRAGMENTS

DAMIAN ROGERS

ALFRED A. KNOPF CANADA

For the mothers
and the daughters
and the dudes

The thing is to join the current
in the depths.

—CLAES OLDENBURG,
ARTIST'S NOTEBOOK

. . . at the end of the story, we will
know more than we know now.

—HANS CHRISTIAN ANDERSEN,
"THE SNOW QUEEN"

But will my heart be broken
when the night meets the
morning sun?

—GERRY GOFFIN & CAROLE KING,
"WILL YOU STILL LOVE ME TOMORROW"

CONTENTS

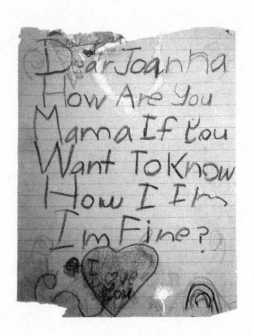

PART I

eagle / earnings / earrings / earthquake / easel
eccentricity / echo / echolalia / eclipse / economy
ecosystem / ecstasy / edge / edification / education
effacement / effectiveness / efficiencies / effort
eggs / egress / egret / ejection / elasticity / elation
elder / elective / electricity / elegy / element
elevator / eligibility / elimination / elision
elitism / ellipsis / elocution / elopement
emanation / emancipation / embarrassment
ember / embodiment / embroidery / emergency
emotion / empiricism / emulation / emulsion
encaustic / enchantment / endearment
endlessness / enigma / enmeshment / envelopes
environment / envy / epigenetics / episode
equality / erasure / eros / erosion / error
escalation / E S C A P E / eternity / evacuation
examination / exclusion / exhaustion / exit
exposure / expulsion / extremities / eye

I MAKE MY life with my mother into a story, and the story makes me.

When my mother, Joanna, escaped from the locked dementia unit at her under-resourced nursing home in Buffalo, I was far away in Toronto, oblivious. I'd fallen asleep early that night, and I stayed asleep until morning. I slept through the call the facility made to my landline after the police brought my mother back around midnight. The nursing home management had waited until she was found to tell me she'd vanished. As a result, I didn't know she was in danger until she was out of it. When I finally talked to the nursing home, nobody there could explain to me how Joanna had managed to make a break into the night on her own. I still don't know what happened to her in those hours she wandered outside by herself. All I can do is imagine.

Although I know it is an impossible fantasy, I imagine an alternate reality in which she had planned her adventure for weeks. I imagine that she'd monitored those who monitored her, waiting for the moment when she might slip out. I imagine that she'd carefully chosen her clothes that day; that she had braided her long brown hair into a smooth inch-thick rope that hung down the centre of her back. In my mind's eye, I dress her in the soft blue cotton sweatshirt my husband, Mike, wouldn't let me buy her at Target, the one that read WEEKEND WANDERER. ("That's really inappropriate," he'd told me when I pulled it off the sale rack.) In my imagination, Joanna walks the streets of Buffalo at midnight feeling no fear. I see her smile at the sensation of cool air on her face, I see her eyes focused and alert to the world around her as she moves freely through space.

I have no way of knowing if Joanna enjoyed her brief break from institutional life, or whether she was frightened, aware immediately that she was lost in a completely unfamiliar landscape. Since arriving at the home, she'd only left the building when escorted to her appointments at a neurology clinic. I do know that the police found her in the parking lot of a Sunoco gas station eight blocks away from the nursing home, two hours after the staff at the facility realized they'd misplaced her between their scheduled checks. It remains a mystery why the alarm system didn't go off when she left. She wore a wander guard around her ankle that never came off; it made a squarish lump under her socks. It looked like a blocky plastic watch from the eighties, except that its smooth grey face did not tell time. The wander guard should have triggered the alarm when Joanna stepped onto the elevator that took her from the fourth floor down to the main floor. It should have set off an alarm when she walked through the nursing home's front door.

When the police approached Joanna, she returned with them to the facility without complaint. My fantasy of her self-determination dissolves here. In reality, she was incapable of even the simplest form of planning. Perhaps she had followed a visiting family onto the elevator and out the door. She looked young, hardly a strand of grey in her uncombed hair. I imagine her more accurately in pyjama pants, no coat in the mid-March chill, wearing slip-on shoes. Was she wearing shoes? I hope she was wearing shoes. I picture her reaching the parking lot, swaying slightly, unsure of her next move. The gas station with its twenty-four-hour food mart selling chips and lottery tickets was one of the only businesses in the neighbourhood. It makes sense to me that she would have been easily guided into a police car. There was nowhere else to go.

A nurse checked Joanna's body for signs of trauma and found no bruises, no abrasions. As she changed Joanna out of her damp clothes, the nurse joked with her. "You decided to take a little walk! How did you get out of the building?"

"Door. Door," my mother muttered, lying down on her bed and turning her back on the woman, who was not so much younger than she was. "I'm tired."

I am able to imagine my mother, and in my imagination I fill the holes in the stories of what happened to her. There are so many holes in the stories, and I am always filling those holes. When I shut my eyes and think of Joanna, she is there. I am able to see her as she was when I visited her last week, as she was two years ago, ten years ago, thirty. I used to feel that I knew the contents of her mind almost as well as the contents of my own. In some ways, that was an illusion, of course; she kept secrets I'll never know. But I understood her moods, the shadows that moved through her, and I knew her heart—what would please her, what would cause her to scowl or clench her jaw. I am still able to reach her, but she drifts further and further away as her illness progresses. I picture her mind as a large dark field filled with a flickering network of rapidly dimming lights. When I imagine her alone in the dark, that night three years ago, I wonder where she was trying to go. I wonder if she was trying to find me.

❦

MANY MONTHS BEFORE Joanna's short escape, I stayed at a friend's empty house in Buffalo, and visited my mother at the nursing home every day for a week. Each day I dropped down deeper inside her world. On my second visit, we retreated to her shared room. Her roommate wasn't there. Beside Joanna's single bed stood the last surviving piece of the bedroom set she'd inherited from her mother, an antique dresser topped with a bevelled-edged mirror in a curving walnut frame. I'd arranged for this to be used instead of the bland dresser issued with the room. There was a brass keyhole in the top drawer, but if there had ever been a corresponding key, it had been lost years ago.

Joanna sat on her bed and examined a wall-mounted fluorescent light fixture, running her fingertips over the bubbled texture of its yellowed plastic shade. She gestured toward it, invited me to appreciate its enigmatic power. "I like this," she said.

I faced her in a chair I'd dragged in from the TV area across from the elevators. I'd positioned a meal tray so that it was between us, an improvised work space. I'd covered its surface with an array of coloured markers and two pages torn from a sketchbook.

When I'd visited the day before, there hadn't been any photos on her side of the room, but now I noticed she had found and propped up three pictures on her dresser. There was a framed photo of my son, Levi, that I'd given her for Christmas four years earlier, when he was a newborn, and there were two loose snapshots. One was of the base of the Eiffel Tower, which Joanna had taken during our weekend trip to Paris together in 1994. The other photo was of me.

I picked up this last picture and studied it. I'm sitting by myself on the blue-and-green floral couch in our living room in suburban Detroit. I'm probably fifteen years old. I'm wearing a baggy acrylic sweater and my hair is pulled back against my head on the sides, a big puff of curled bangs clawing at my eyebrows. Everything in this photo now looked ugly to me: my clothes, the pink walls behind me, the purple calico-print tablecloth on the side table, that awful couch, the ruffled muslin curtains my grandmother had made for us, just like the ones in her own house.

Joanna leaned forward, her soft, plump arm touching mine, and she too looked at the photo in my hands.

"You're my beautiful baby," she said. I kissed her cheek.

The room was dark. I crossed to the window over her roommate's bed and pulled the fraying cord to raise the blinds. I sat down on the edge of the mattress and looked out through a tangle of bare tree branches to the street below.

Joanna had followed me over, and she stood behind me as we looked out the window silently for a moment. Then she pointed across the street and said, "You see that thing there . . ."

"I'm not sure what you're pointing at, the houses or the cars parked on the street?"

Her dark brows drew together. "I don't know," she said, and turned away from the window.

We settled back on her side of the room, sitting again with the meal tray I'd set up between us. I used the little speaker on my phone to stream the Beatles record she owned when I was little, back when we lived with my grandparents. It was the only record she had salvaged from the two years she lived in California before I was born.

"What colour marker do you want to use first?" I asked her. She hesitated and then pointed to purple, looking back up at me for reassurance. "Oh, that's a great choice," I said.

My mother held the marker awkwardly, looking down at it uncertainly.

"Here, I'm going to draw a circle on the page like this, and you can colour it in," I said as I drew a wobbly round blob.

"Oh, you're doing such a good job," she said.

After some hesitation, she slowly started to make short purple strokes along the inside of the circle. I continued to praise her as I drew a cluster of triangles and dots on my own page. After a while, she stopped moving her hand to watch mine.

"Yours is so beautiful," she said.

"So is yours," I told her, but I couldn't redirect her attention back to her own page. "Here, we'll draw this together," I told her, putting my own drawing away in my bag.

My phone played one of the Beatles' many hits from the year she went to see the band play Olympia Stadium in Detroit with her girlfriends. That was the year she turned fifteen. She'd told me about that show, how she couldn't hear a single note they

sang, the music drowned out by the sounds of the girls screaming around her. We sang along—"She loves you and you know
that can't be bad"—as our heads bent toward each other over
the purple ring Joanna had made in the centre of the page.
I added a black dot in the middle of the ring, then drew round
petals around the perimeter, making a psychedelic flower with
a cartoonish eye at its centre.

"Oh, that's nice," she said.

I continued to draw on her page, asking her to choose
colours for me. "We'll do this together," I said again. "We're
collaborating."

I adjusted my sense of time as we sang and I drew, listening
to the whole double album with the door shut. We dropped out
of time and space. We were the only two people in the world.
We were alone at the bottom of an ocean.

Someone knocked and the door opened. It was John, a man
I'd met the day before in front of the nurses' station, beside the
TV. He had told me he loved me as he shook my hand. He had
the red face, bright-blue eyes and silver brush cut I associate with
Midwestern football coaches. Like Joanna, he was wearing
loose-fitting elastic-waist pants and fuzzy socks with no-slip
strips. No shoes.

"Oh, hi!" he said, lighting up as he saw me. "What are you
girls doing?"

"Oh, we're just spending time together," I said lightly, and
looked back down at the drawing.

"I told you yesterday that I loved you," he said.

This guy, I thought, and kept drawing.

"This is my baby," my mother said, her hand on my arm. "Isn't
she beautiful?"

"Yes, I told you that yesterday," John said. He turned his square body to me again. His eyes glinted in the flat fluorescent light. "Can I kiss you?" He was blocking the door.

"Nope," I said with a big smile.

He smiled too. "Okay, I won't do anything you don't want. But I love to see you. Why don't you visit more?"

I winced. "I live in Canada," I told him.

"Oh," he said, satisfied. "When are you coming back?"

"Soon," I said. "I'll be back soon."

"Okay, you come see me. I love your mother, but I really love seeing you." He winked. "I'll leave you girls alone now."

Joanna and I returned to our own zone again, but the spell was soon broken by screams on the other side of the door. My mother was not disturbed; she seemed to not hear the noise at all. I pretended I needed to go to the bathroom as an excuse to open the door and look out . . .

"You can just go to this one in here," Joanna said, pointing to the bathroom between her room and the one next door.

"Um, okay, I just want to—" I poked my head out. I could hear a fight, but I couldn't see a thing. "It's okay, I'm fine," I said, pulling my head in and shutting the door again.

When I opened the door an hour later to walk to the elevator with my mother, a woman of indeterminate age sat on the floor in front of me. This is a horror movie, I thought; this is the nineteenth century. The previous year, when Joanna had first moved from a nice assisted-living facility into this run-down nursing home, the only thing she'd said to me was, "There are a lot of people suffering here." She had always been sensitive to the pain of those around her. Not long after this, she lost the ability to speak in complete, coherent sentences.

Her current home was the only place that would take her when the assisted-living facility pushed her out of their system—a system I'd chosen for their well-maintained buildings, for their reputation for keeping residents in their care after savings ran out and they transitioned to Medicaid. But my mother's diagnosis of frontal-lobe dementia had made her an unattractive resident. *Inappropriate* was the word they used when they first approached me about finding her a new place to live. "She's an inappropriate resident."

I opened the door from our pocket of calm and saw a woman whose hands were wrapped around the doorknob of the room across the hall from us. The woman was hunched down on the floor with her knees pressed to her chest, the weight of her small, wiry body hanging from her grip on the doorknob. Our eyes locked and she began to sob. As my mother and I passed her, she stood up and followed us, asking for help, trying to get my attention. Joanna muttered, "Just ignore her," as we inched sideways, gripping each other's forearms, toward the elevator.

❦

IN 2010, SIX MONTHS before I knew Joanna was sick, we had been drinking herbal tea in her new living room in the Buffalo suburbs as she told me about the young adult fantasy novel she was writing. The story follows a brother and sister, born in exile, as they search the galaxies in a time machine for their ancestral planet, a home they've never seen. They attend classes at the School of the Crystal Caves. They play games with their companion animal, a creature called a *mercasa*. They meet Aden of the Starlit Mountains and visit the Treehouses of Odysseus.

"I've always been an escapist," Joanna said with a smirk.

This is a talent I inherited from her. Over the years, I have found so many different ways to escape, to disappear: depression, performance, alcohol, panic, work. Leaving my body is a familiar sensation, although I rarely consciously observe it; instead, my awareness draws upwards, collecting in my head, where the pressure soon becomes unbearable. My breathing changes, I overload, I crave a system shutdown. But now I know, if I'm going to survive this—my mother's illness, my many failures in the face of it—it will be through learning how to resist the impulse to evacuate. To learn how to stay here.

I'm aware that this idea of inheritance scares me. In one of the back rooms of my brain, I struggle to draw a line between my mother's life and my own.

Part of me now, as I write this, is still there on the fourth floor of the nursing home, waiting for the elevator beside Joanna. We stood there, pretending not to see the woman crying next to us, waiting. When the doors finally opened and I jumped onto the elevator, my mother had to take a couple steps back so that she was far enough from the doors that her wander guard didn't set off the alarm. It took a long time for those doors to shut. I kept telling Joanna that I loved her as I held down the Close Doors button, waving goodbye, good night, sweet dreams, until the doors slowly slid between us and I descended.

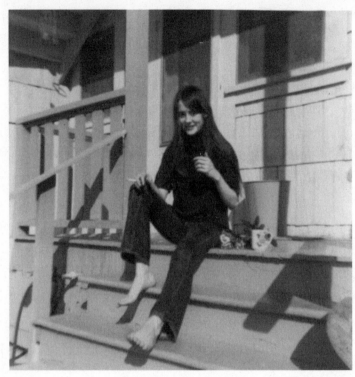

JOANNA, 1970
Unknown porch in Long Beach, California
Unknown photographer

jab / jabber / jacket / jackhammer / Jacuzzi
jade / jaguar / jail / jammies / J A N U A R Y
jasmine / jasper / jay / jealousy / jeans / jellyfish
jeopardy / jeremiad / jet / jewel / jezebel
jigsaw / jinx / jitters / jobs / joint / jokes / jolt
journal / journey / joy / judgment / juice
jumble / jump-cut / juncture / jury / justice
justification / juvenile / juxtaposition

up baby bottle

donnie's breakfast

mine—

baby nap—dishes—/
also living room. letters
on alternate wk.

feed baby. relax—

clean bedroom

JOANNA'S ZIPPERED
NOTEBOOK, 1972

WHEN I WAS a baby, Joanna kept a four-inch-by-seven-inch, olive-green, faux leather zippered notebook in which she documented her domestic ambitions. The first four pages are filled with ideas for decorating the apartment she was sharing with my father and me in a faltering neighbourhood in downtown Detroit. After the notes on *furniture ideas* such as *refinish picnic tables for kitchen*, the following four pages are devoted to planning meals—not recipes, simply lists of various dishes, grouped under categories and subheadings: *Main courses: Homemade Soups—vegetable, potato, chicken, corn. Vegetables: Corn—cob, creamed, plain; Carrots—cooked with butter, plain, cooked with orange juice and brown sugar. Salads: Tossed; Cottage Cheese; Fruit; Coleslaw; Jello.* After the menu plans, there is a page with the subject heading "baby": *Toys—xmas & birthday, decoupage blocks, make blue velvet dress, make pooh animals, make colorful cloth books, pull toys, doll.* There is an emphatically underlined directive to self: _REGULARLY: Make beads out of empty spools, paint and decoupage, string & elastic. Make a small doll collection._ There is also a schedule for how she should organize her days.

I didn't know my father when I was growing up, although he lived with my mother and me for the first year of my life. The clearest vision I have of this time emerges from these notes Joanna kept, which I braid together with the rare, brief stories she'd told me when I was young, and with what my father remembers now, more than four decades later.

The notebook holds a spooky power for me. The blue ballpoint pen she used to make the notes is still nestled inside the six tiny silver spirals that bind the custom-sized, tightly lined paper. Inside an inner plastic flap, I found a name and address written on part of a brown paper napkin, and a folded piece of typing paper with a list of _Beauty Aids: Ideas etc._ (They are written as imperatives: _Wash face with nail brush & soap in shower for complete rinse. When can afford liquid blusher mix with baby lotion or cream. Invest in baby powder, light blue eyeshadow, beige/peach lipstick. Use perfume liber-ally._) The small zippered notebook is a talisman; I feel as if I can talk back to the person who is writing—has written—these things down. On one page she makes notes for drawings she wants to do:

Wind—fall. Snow Queen—winter. Sun—summer. Spring?

Flowers, I want to tell her, make flowers for spring. Or rain.

Also in the notebook's inner plastic pocket: three paper fair-ies, cut free from the pages of a children's magazine.

❦

JOANNA TOLD ME almost nothing about my missing father. I sniffed out fresh details every time I asked her who he was, and where he was.

"Maybe he's dead," I said one day.

"He's not dead," she answered.

"Well," I said. "He could be." As far as I could see, he had disappeared into the void.

"He's not dead," she repeated. She seemed uneasy. I let it drop.

They'd divorced when I was two weeks old, my mother told me whenever I asked. I asked a lot.

"It had nothing to do with you," she assured me once, although it had never occurred to me that it had.

Piecing their story together has been a lifelong project. What I did eventually learn: My father met Joanna when she was in crisis. My father, with whom I reconnected in adulthood, doesn't remember the season, and Joanna no longer remembers my father, so precision isn't available to me. I only know that one day in 1970 she knocked on the door of his apartment in Long Beach, California. He'd grown up in that neighbourhood, and his mother and sisters still lived nearby. Joanna had moved to their Long Beach neighbourhood the previous year from the Detroit suburbs.

Though he was only twenty, my father lived alone in a former military building across the street from the Dow Chemical Plant. Joanna was selling Avon cosmetics door to door, and it was a short walk through the industrial park from the apartment where she was living with her husband and his best friend.

What my father remembers best about his first meeting with Joanna is that she was "a fine-looking woman," that she was "model-esque." He also said she looked like she might be starving. What my mother remembered best, in the years before her illness, was that my father answered the door with a sandwich in his hand. There was no food in her apartment. She *was* starving.

I have a photograph of Joanna from that year, and she looks like a child swimming in hand-me-downs. She wore her hair straight, with long bangs that framed her large brown eyes. She was almost twenty-one but could still easily pass for a teenager.

My father invited her in for coffee and they talked for a while. Usually, there was not enough time in a day for Joanna to drink coffee. My father had asthma, but I always imagine he let her smoke that day. She used to hold her cigarette between her third and fourth fingers, like a European, and her hands were always moving when she spoke. She told me once about a guy she dated who insisted she wouldn't be able to speak if he held her hands down, and then restrained her to prove it. I recall exasperated fury lifting off her skin as she told me about it. When she sat in my father's apartment for the first time, what did the two of them talk about? My father was four months younger than Joanna, an age difference he never forgot to mention, as if they were on different timelines.

Did she tell him right away that she was married? I imagine she did, explaining how she'd moved to California from Michigan the year before with her husband and his friend.

"So, if I buy something, you'll have to come back?" This is what my father says he asked. I imagine his desire for my mother in his face and voice.

"Yes, I guess I will." This is what my father says she replied. I imagine her smiling.

❦

I CAN MAKE the story only by alternating between the fragments my mother and my father separately told me over the years. Joanna's stories started earlier in my life, but were always guarded and brief. And they changed, sometimes opening up to include a new piece of information, or a hint at the emotional currents beneath. Other times, the narrative would abruptly dissolve to black: The End. She was always pulling a screen between me and her past, and I was always working to find a way to see behind the screen.

She had told me how she had followed her boyfriend to California in 1969, a couple years after she'd graduated from high school, where they'd met. He'd bought her a razor before they were married, a gift her parents found distasteful. (She was still using that razor when I was in high school; it was the one I used when I started to shave my own legs.) I imagine what future they might have dreamed of together, what kind of life they'd planned for themselves in Los Angeles. Joanna wanted to be an artist; I have no idea what he wanted to be. He had headed to Los Angeles with his friend first, and my mother joined them once they'd found an apartment. My father told me she'd said she'd liked the sound of Long Beach when her future-husband mentioned the neighbourhood over the phone. I doubt she had pictured the chemical plants.

After Joanna met up with her boyfriend in California, a mail-order minister married them in a private ceremony on the beach. Whenever I asked my mother about the past, she liked to reference the period details of her wedding: blue jeans, wildflowers, love beads, sunset.

What exactly happened to the three of them—Joanna, her husband, his friend—is not clear to me. I do know that, whatever it was, it was bad. My mother hinted throughout my childhood that she had lost herself in some way, and that she didn't really understand what had happened to her during this time. Doctors she saw afterward, she told me, suggested she had sustained a closed head injury, an injury she couldn't remember or name. She confessed to me once that for a time she had thought she was in love with the friend who was living with them. She described this as an episode of amnesia, a kind of psychosis, said that she didn't remember who she was, or *whose* she was.

By the time she ended up at my father's apartment with an Avon catalogue, she was no longer sleeping with her husband but still felt a sense of responsibility toward him. Or that's what she told me. Her stories changed slightly over the years, although some details were repeated many times. But I now understand that doesn't mean they are true.

❧

IN MY FATHER'S version, Joanna returned weeks after their first meeting to deliver the Snoopy cologne decanter that my father had ordered. She was changed, he said. She had lost more weight, looked even more fragile, emaciated, hollow-eyed. My father invited her in again and she opened up to him. Her husband, she said, was covering the windows with aluminum foil, and had unplugged the radio because he thought it was bugged. He'd accused her of trying to control his heartbeat with her breath. "They were getting into dark energies, all three of them," my father told me. "Aleister Crowley–type stuff."

Joanna didn't know anyone else in Long Beach, didn't have money or anywhere to go. So my father invited her to stay with him. "She was in a bad situation," he told me. "She was in distress. I guess I liked the idea of saving her."

My father had grown up surfing in Long Beach. He had blue eyes, long dark hair, a naturally pale complexion that was deeply tanned from his time in the sun. He had a job working at Monsanto, stacking fifty-pound bags of chemicals. The rumour on the floor was that the bags were being sent to the American War in Vietnam. "But we didn't really know," he told me.

His job paid well and made it possible for my father to cover his own rent and to own a motorcycle and two other vehicles. He and a friend painted his 1962 Pontiac Grand Prix low-rider so that it looked black but then glowed violet and blue when the light hit it just right. "Blue Murano Pearl—it was cutting-edge paint technology," he told me. "We would cruise down Bellflower Boulevard and the girls would whistle." He also owned a converted milk truck that he used like a dune buggy at the beach. He had a curious mind and read widely, favouring visionary novels by Hermann Hesse, Kurt Vonnegut and J.R.R. Tolkien, as well as books on esoteric subjects, like reincarnation. Raised Irish Catholic, he was fascinated by the story of Father Damien, a missionary from Belgium who rebelled against his superiors in order to minister to those dying in the Hawaiian leprosy colony of Molokai.

❦

MY PARENTS SPENT one Christmas together in California. Joanna told me how strange it was to think of Santa sailing over palm trees. She remembered seeing a plastic sleigh pulled by seahorses on a neighbour's roof. She also told me that my father's mother handed her a glass of eggnog with so much rum in it my mother felt as if she might slide to the floor after one sip. Joanna was pretty straight. "Her drugs of choice were coffee and cigarettes," my father confirmed much later.

When my father worked the night shift, Joanna would stay up all night waiting for him, drinking coffee, smoking cigarettes and drawing. When he worked the day shift, she would visit with his mother or his sisters.

They may have been living in Los Angeles, but my father's neighbourhood had a small-town quality to it. It turned out a woman my father knew from high school was dating Joanna's husband's friend, the one who had lived with Joanna and her husband. This woman reached out to my father through a note. "There are things you should know," she'd said in it, inviting him to coffee.

But when my father told my mother about this, she became distraught. "She made it clear it would be an unforgivable betrayal if I went," he told me. "So I didn't go. But I always wondered what it was she wanted to tell me about. I got the sense that maybe your mother had gone a little crazy. Maybe they *all* had gone a little crazy."

❧

FROM WHAT I can gather, my parents lived together for about a year in California. During that time, Joanna became pregnant and miscarried. The doctors told her she couldn't have a baby. She was too skinny.

My parents fought. They went to couples counselling once or twice. At some point the therapist took my father aside and said, "It's really important you keep coming back. There's a lot going on here."

But Joanna said no. "I don't need my head shrunk," she insisted.

❦

MY FATHER EVENTUALLY sent Joanna home to her parents for good. He'd already tried this several times. "It wasn't working," he said.

"I was very fond of her," he told me. "I cared for her. Was I in love with her? I don't know."

It was too much responsibility, he said. He had just turned twenty-one. Let someone else look after her. He left things open-ended, but he didn't really want her back. She was needy, unemployed. His friends didn't like that she flirted with them, and told him so. "She was very sensual," he said, "in everything she did—the way she smoked, the way she walked down the street . . . And she seemed to think having a baby would be this wonderful experience," he said through his teeth.

❦

JOANNA ARRIVED BACK in Michigan in April 1971.

Her older sister, my aunt, once told me, "Before you were born, Mom said, 'Jo's come back from California really crazy.' She denied that she was pregnant, but she was clearly showing."

Joanna told me many times that she had gained twenty-four pounds when she was pregnant with me, "the perfect amount." She barely weighed a hundred pounds to start. She had such a small frame, her belly must have been hard to hide.

She wrote my father a love letter begging him to visit but not revealing the urgency. He decided to come in September, to meet her people and see what autumn looked like in Michigan. They were on the phone finalizing details when she suddenly said, "My mother says I should tell you I'm pregnant."

"I guess you don't want to come now," she added.

"You're damn right I don't!" my father told her. He did the math. She was at least five months pregnant. If the child was his.

"I was upset," he told me.

But his own mother told him he should go.

❧

I HOLD IN my mind two significantly different versions of a conversation between my grandfather and my father, when my father was in Michigan for those ten days in September.

In Joanna's version, my grandfather told my father not to come back if he wasn't prepared to marry Joanna.

In my father's version, my grandfather said this, yes, but then he also said, "Look, if you want to try to make this work, we will do everything we can to support you. But if it doesn't work, do Joanna a favour and don't hang around so that she holds on to hope. Let her move on."

"I was confused," my father told me. "The whole situation really was a shock."

Months after that conversation, my father left California on New Year's Day 1972, slowly driving his unheated modified milk truck through the Southern states, postponing his turn north for as long as possible. He slept in the truck at night, snuggled up to an Irish setter named Shaughnessy, running the engine when the cold was unbearable. No one in my mother's family was sure when to expect him. Joanna often told me that I'd shown up exactly on my due date. I don't think she fully believed my father would show up at all.

❦

IT WAS MY grandmother who took my mother to the hospital— my grandmother who, according to my father, had months earlier noted that Joanna "waited too long to do anything about it."

At the hospital, Joanna shared a room with a married woman who had just had a miscarriage. Joanna was aware of this woman watching as my mother held me in her arms for the first time. She said the woman couldn't take her eyes off me. The point of this story, I knew, was to praise me for being valued, desirable: beautiful. But the story was also about my mother's perception of this woman's envy—what my mother interpreted as the woman's hope that she, Joanna, was a troubled teen looking to give up her child for adoption.

"And how old are you?" the woman had asked her. When she told me this, Joanna always imitated the patronizing lilt in the woman's voice, the high-pitched tone people use when speaking to children or animals.

"Twenty-two," Joanna had said, meeting her gaze.

"I could tell the woman thought I was around fourteen years old," she told me, her eyes narrowed and her lips curled slightly. "I could tell she wanted you."

In my mind, Joanna held me tightly. *Mine.*

❧

THE FACT THAT my parents weren't married to each other was a source of deep shame for my mother's family. Because Joanna had been married before she met my father and was in fact still legally married when I was born, she was counselled at the hospital to name her husband as my father, even though she hadn't seen him in well over nine months. When Joanna explained this subterfuge tearfully to me when I was ten, I imagined a panel of impartial legal advisers who wanted only to protect me from the harsh judgment of an unfair world. But thinking about it now, as an adult, I realize it was probably my grandmother who did the counselling. My grandmother was the one who accompanied Joanna to the hospital when she went into labour. And my grandmother was keenly invested in the judgment of the world.

When my father arrived the following day, he discovered that his name wasn't on the birth certificate.

❦

THE YEAR OF MY BIRTH was also the year my father first experienced winter. Among the photos of me as a newborn that he took in that first month of 1972 are several street scenes, showing the snow pressing down on my grandparents' small house in suburban Detroit. They had already lived inside that three-bedroom, one-bathroom bungalow for nearly twenty years; they raised four kids in that house. The streets were lined with long, clunky, hard-angled cars. My grandfather had worked for Pontiac, and so this was the only make of vehicle in the driveway.

For six months we all lived with my grandparents: Joanna, my father, me and Shaughnessy. Later my mother would roll her eyes and say, "He showed up at my parents' house with a dog that wasn't housebroken."

My father told me, "Shaughnessy was a great travelling companion because he didn't talk much, he just listened."

In their three-bedroom house, my grandparents each had their own room. My mother and I occupied the third, and my father was relegated to the basement. He told me that Joanna would sneak downstairs at night to visit him.

After six months, my father got a job in an auto factory and my parents and I moved into our own apartment near 7 Mile. My father described it as "a neighbourhood in decline." To illustrate this, my mother, who barely spoke of that time to me, once told me a story about a night when a man would not stop pounding on their door. She described him as a giant man, white, dressed like a biker. Joanna was home alone and the door to the apartment was at the bottom of a steep flight of stairs. The man yelled and yelled at her to open the door, and Joanna slowly made her way down the stairs and slid the dead-bolt chain into its track, only a window of glass between her and the red-faced man, who grew louder and angrier by the moment. Then she ran upstairs and waited, terrified, for my father to come home.

For years after, Joanna had nightmares about trying to lock her door while someone banged on the other side, only to then realize that part of the wall behind her was missing, exposing her completely.

❦

THAT SUMMER, MY father's two sisters visited Detroit. His older sister, my aunt Gina, brought her baby, born three months after me. Gina later admitted that she was scandalized to see Joanna pour Hi-C into my bottle. "I wasn't going to let anything like that go inside *my* baby," she told me.

My aunts visited a public garden and took the only photo of me and my parents that I've ever seen. My mother sits cradling me in her arms, and my father stands beside her, his arm around her shoulder. Whichever aunt took the photograph stood at a distance in order to include rows of red and yellow flowers surrounding us. My parents aren't smiling. Their expressions are blurry, but even so, my father's jaw looks clenched, Joanna's face melancholy, her mouth slack, her whole spirit pointing toward the earth. At least, this is how I see it in my mind. Somewhere, somehow, I lost that photo.

❧

A STORY MY mother liked to tell:

My father sat in a chair and called out to my mother, "Bring me a beer!"

She pulled a can out of the fridge and, as she walked, she shook it in short, tight movements against her leg so he couldn't see what she was doing. She handed it to him, and he opened the beer, and of course it sprayed all over him. "He yelled and yelled, and I just laughed."

❧

THE WORKING CONDITIONS at my father's auto plant were unsafe, and some workers started passing around a piece of paper for people to sign if they were interested in unionizing. My father signed it. The next day, everyone whose name was on that piece of paper—about thirty men—was fired.

"Your mom left me that same week," he told me.

Joanna's story of this time was different. My father kept leaving and then returning to their apartment in Detroit, she said, and this made it impossible for her to qualify for government assistance, which she had hated applying for in the first place. He'd be gone, she told me, and she would apply for Aid to Families with Dependent Children, and then he'd come back for a while and she would be denied assistance.

When my dad lost his job, everything unravelled quickly. My aunt talked my grandparents into allowing Joanna and me to move back into their house. What would have happened if my grandparents hadn't taken us in? My parents were losing their apartment. Joanna would have had to find a place to live; she would have had to collect welfare. Joanna felt a shame in this, and she was aware that landlords didn't want to rent to single mothers. I wonder what offices she may have taken me to, what lines we may have waited in, when I was already walking, crying, wanting to be home, to play. Did she ever leave me with a neighbour? She would have had no community. She would have been alone.

If my mother was alone, my father was even more isolated. My father, living through the ugly Detroit winter, unemployed, with no family, no real friends.

My father was relieved when Joanna and I moved back in with my grandparents. Joanna wasn't able to keep up any kind of structure for me outside her parents' home, he said.

"If it makes you feel any better," he told me, "I was glad to be out from under the weight of the relationship with your mom, but heartbroken at losing you."

MY FATHER SOON found a job near Ann Arbor, about forty-five minutes away, working security at an institution for the criminally insane. He moved to the area, and pretty soon after that he had a new girlfriend.

That spring, he visited with his camera and took a roll of film of me. In these photos I am in dirty hand-me-downs, looking up at him. Smiling at the front door, looking up at him. Standing on the brick path in my grandparents' still-barren backyard, looking up at him. On a swing at the nearby tot lot, looking up at him from between two thick links of chain, Joanna's brass-buttoned suede coat behind me, her head cut off.

❦

THE LAST TIME I saw my father during my early childhood was three months later. There had been no visits in between. My mother told me that he had brought along a copy of the self-help paperback *I'm OK—You're OK*, plus the change from the five-dollar bill he'd used to buy it. "That was his idea of child support," she said.

Joanna gave him an ultimatum. "I thought he was just going to screw you up if he swooped in every few months. I told him to visit you regularly, and pay seventy-five dollars a month in child support, or forget it." This is a story she told me many times. That number has never left my head.

My father made his choice. He has since told me that he never forgot me, but at the time I was only a year and a half old. I forgot him.

In my father's version, he arranged to take me to the zoo, and Joanna assumed she would be coming too. At the last minute she realized that he planned to take me to the zoo with his new girlfriend. Joanna was enraged; the zoo was cancelled. When he arrived for the visit, my grandmother went to her room and slammed the door behind her, refusing to speak to him. "It was pretty hostile," he told me.

Though my father is the only person left now whom I can ask about my past, and though I know my mother was always an inconsistent narrator, I still naturally lean into her version. I'm glad to have the other details my father is able to give me, but my sympathies remain with the one who stuck around. I am loyal to the one who was loyal to me.

❧

IT'S HARD TO SAY how much we are shaped by what we can't remember. My mother told me I stopped speaking for a while after she and my father split up. When I started speaking again, I began with new words. I wonder, was this when she moved in with my grandparents in January, a week before my first birthday? Or was it after the last time I saw him, when I was eighteen months old?

❧

JOANNA DID MAKE me those building blocks she'd mentioned in her notebook. My grandfather cut pieces of wood with the power saw in his basement workshop and my mother shellacked illustrations she'd cut out of books onto each one. On one, the Snow Queen beckoned to me with her chilly glamour, her long limbs extending out from under an enormous ermine coat, her long face adorned with diamonds, the black arms of winter trees scratching the sky behind her. Joanna always pointed out the beauty of the winter trees on our suburban streets. "They look like ink drawings," she'd say.

In my grandparents' house, Joanna drank coffee and watched me play with my blocks on the floor.

❦

DURING OUR LAST Christmas together in that apartment in Detroit, Joanna wrote a short story in the back of her zippered notebook about a tiny magical man who emerged from the forest to sneak up on the bad little children who had grown up and pretended very hard to be good. Crossed out at the top of the following page was "and everyone was happy, even the cynical." Beneath the scribble over this, I can see that she had corrected "was happy" to read "*is* happy."

It was January 1973 when Joanna left that apartment where the three of us had lived for six months. No daddy now, no dog. Joanna left behind her little zippered notebook, and my father kept it for forty years. Only then did he give it to me, along with a box containing all the letters my mother and I had ever

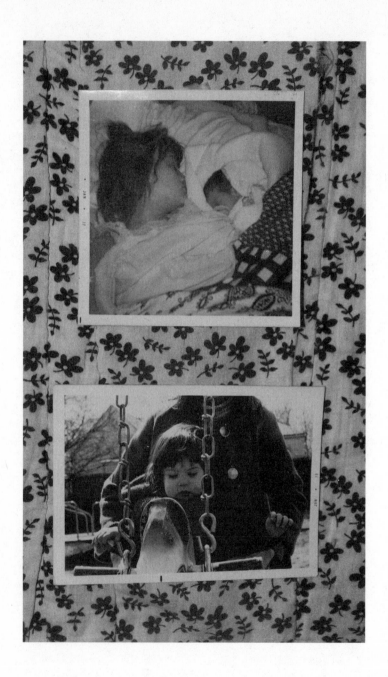

written him. Inside the notebook are her hopes to build a home. The last legible words in the little zippered notebook read:

> *And the snowflakes*
> *said to one another*
>
> *that sometimes people*
> *were almost human.*

After that: twenty blank pages.

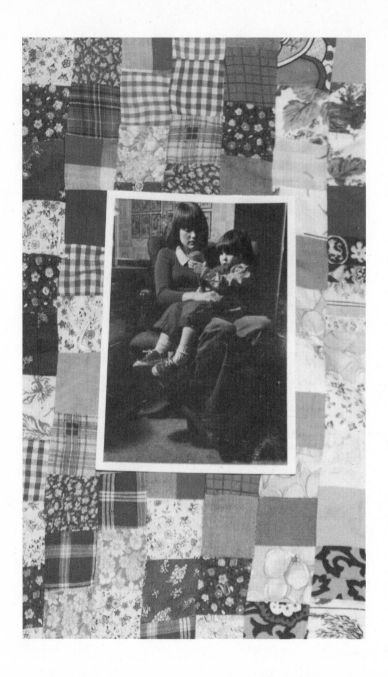

quaintness / qualification / quality / qualms
quandary / quantity / quarrel / quartz
quatrain / quaver / queasiness / queen
querulousness / query / quest / questions / quid
quiet / quill / Q U I L T / quintessence / quip
quirk / quitter / quiver / quote / quotient

I stood at
the top of
the stairs
and called

Jo-Jo!
Up Jo-Jo!

Up!

Joanna tired on her bed
in the basement

IN THE BASEMENT, Joanna is talking to herself, and I am sitting at the top of the stairs, listening.

My earliest memories are of reaching out for my mother. I called her Jo-Jo before I called her Mama, because I listened to my grandparents call her Jo. Whenever I was upset, I cried, "I want my Jo-Jo!" After eating breakfast with my grandfather at the table—grapefruit juice, Grape-Nuts covered in sugar—I'd stand at the top of the back stairs and call down to the basement, where she slept in a makeshift bedroom, "Up, Jo-Jo, up!" I remember standing at the bottom of a stepladder set up beneath the apple tree in the backyard as she dropped hard green fruit into a metal bucket beside me. I remember the leaves, and her jeans, her bare feet.

Though there are many photographs of my mother and me, in my earliest memories she's not there. She's missing. She's asleep, or she's in another room, or she's at work, or out of the house with her boyfriend. I wander through the house in search of her.

I sat on the stairs that led to the basement, out of her view, and listened to her talk to herself. She sounded as if she was in the middle of a heated argument with an invisible adversary. She paced back and forth, her arms moving through the air in great sweeps of motion.

"Promise me you'll never talk to yourself," she said to me once. "People will think you're crazy."

❦

MY GRANDMOTHER WATCHED me often, and she watched me closely. She collected my drawings, carefully annotating each one, dating them and transcribing my descriptions in quotes.

> *"Bee."*
> *"A talking pear."*
> *"A kitty cat" with "eyes."*
> *"A pretend monster."*

If she wasn't cooking, or sewing, or cleaning, Grandma could almost always be found in her nest, her name for the nook she set up in the corner of the red velvet couch in the living room, where she sat surrounded by books and pillows. She was always making notes inside a spiral notebook. Sometimes I would lie with my head on a pillow in her lap and she would scrape the wax out of my ears with a bobby pin. "Do you clean Grandpa's ears too?" I once asked. She was disgusted by the suggestion that she would touch him in this intimate way.

In the evenings, she drank cream sherry from a wineglass and Grandpa would drink cans of Pabst Blue Ribbon beer. We watched Lawrence Welk on television, where silver-haired singers stood stiffly against a background of baby-blue bubbles. I would play the only record Joanna had salvaged from her time in California, the red Beatles compilation. I was fascinated by the portraits of the band photographed four years apart looking over the same staircase: first boyish, then hairy. I'd stare at the photos of these men, how they were mixed into a crowd peering through the bars of a cage at the zoo, their faces sad, as if they understood how the unseen animals felt to be living on display, in captivity. I'd play other records from the stack behind the television: Frankie Avalon, Mahalia Jackson, Elvis, an early electronic music record called *Switched-On Bach* and the dated comedy stylings of Tom Lehrer. Grandma would play popular songs from her childhood on the piano and I'd watch her feet pumping the pedals, the unnatural flat tan shade of her pantyhose.

When I was four, I taught myself to read. I was frightened by an image in Dr. Seuss's *One Fish Two Fish Red Fish Blue Fish* of a brother and sister carrying an enormous monster trapped in a jar of dark-green water up a flight of stairs. I adored a story I found in a children's book from the 1920s about a neglected boy dying of consumption whose only possession was the piece of the moon that shone in his garret window at night. Joanna hated that story.

"Damy is working away on her reading—I've never seen a child so <u>want</u> to learn," my grandmother wrote in her notebook as she watched from her nest.

What I wanted to learn was how to be more like her.

Once, for weeks, my grandmother sat with her head bent over a wooden embroidery hoop that held a section of pale-blue chambray taut as stretched canvas, the tip of her tongue between her lips, her face focused in concentration on the path of her needle. She was following the outline of images she had asked Joanna to draw on a Western-cut shirt for me. Soon, the yoke and cuffs were covered in shaggy yellow dandelion heads, delicate pale-pink clover blossoms and vibrant-green leaves—the wildflowers of our suburban lawn—all filled in with satin-finish floss. On the pocket, my name in lower-case cursive, Joanna's most careful handwriting, traced in chain stitch right over my heart.

❧

IN THE DINING ROOM, a framed magazine illustration of Tennessee Williams. An antique iron, the kind that had to be heated on the top of a coal-burning stove before it could be used to smooth the creases out of cotton clothes. A miniature cast iron stove. In the corner, my grandmother's sewing machine. She made most of my clothes, the ones that weren't hand-me-downs. In the mornings, I sat with my grandfather, at the table there, eating breakfast and reading the newspaper. A small glass of grapefruit juice. Comics. *Brenda Starr* and *Modesty Blaise*. Every night we all ate dinner together at five o'clock sharp. My grandfather sometimes with a rocks glass by his hand, a little amber liquid at the bottom. Stewed rhubarb, homemade pickles, biscuits, tomato soup, tuna fish and rice. Had I had this before? Did I like it?

THE KITCHEN WAS blue and red. A small orange glass square with an illustration of the herb marjoram painted onto it hung from a thin brown velvet ribbon in front of the window over the sink, catching light. Large jars of dried beans lined the small marble-topped workspace where Grandma made bread, biscuits, chopped vegetables. Every morning, Grandma woke up early and made herself a bacon sandwich and coffee, carefully scraping the grease from the pan into a fat ceramic jar beside the stove. She carried her breakfast down the hall and back into her bedroom on a tray and shut the door. Later she would be back in the kitchen before every meal. Grandma baked bread twice a week, large metal bowls on the marble counter holding balls of dough under damp dishcloths. They swelled like beige puffball mushrooms before being divided into loaf pans, enough for the family and a few favourite neighbours. In the evenings after dinner, Joanna would help Grandma with the dishes, drying each one as it came out of the rinsing sink, and I would throw tantrums, holding on to my mother's ankles and screaming as she sighed.

MY GRANDFATHER'S ROOM was painted pale blue and his royal-blue bedspread had thin raised stripes of a knobby texture, a kind of rough cousin to chenille. Because my grandfather flew small planes as a hobby, my grandmother had papered one of his walls with aeronautical charts, flight planning maps in muted blues, greens and yellows. I was fascinated by the series of circles and blocky shapes that represented the ground as a pilot needs to see it. (He took me up in the air in a rented two-seater on Saturdays, grinned when I pointed out the window at the buildings below and called them "dollhouses." My grandfather was building a dollhouse replica of the farmhouse where my grandmother had been born.) On his desk: a small metal scale for calculating the cost by weight of stamps needed to send a letter by mail. In his desk drawers: rolls of stamps, envelopes, paper clips, a rubber-band ball and a secret cache of Clark candy bars replenished with left-overs every year after Halloween. Beside the bed he kept a framed photo of me in his bed, home one day with the flu, smiling up from behind a magazine, my legs under the covers. In his basement workshop, to the left of the stairs, where I watched him work on the grinding circular saws from a respectful distance, he made miniature furniture, including a replica of his own antique bed, its towering headboard carved with delicate branches.

❦

MY GRANDMOTHER'S ROOM was red and her bed was covered in quilts. She had a vanity and an electric typewriter, pale blue, on which she typed letters to distant family members and light verse about the politics of social square dancing ("Other People in the Set"). On the vanity were an old hairbrush and hand mirror that were decorative only, beside a small tin box from Paris filled with buttons of all different sizes, colours and shapes.

One drawer held the plastic box of her hot rollers and the numerous chiffon scarves she kept to tie around her head when she was wearing the curlers. She kept her jewellery in her dresser: a necklace of natural coral; a heavy brass cross with a Byzantine-style Christ; a silver-and-turquoise eagle, probably bought at a trading post in Montana; and an ivory bracelet carved with elephants that her beloved lost brother had bought for her during the war. A photograph of him in uniform hung beside portraits of each of her two sons wearing sailor hats, my uncles, taken when they went into the navy, two years apart.

❦

THE GREEN-TILED BATHROOM had two mirrored medicine cabinets, a framed Valentine's Day card from the 1920s featuring four different white women with long, flowing hair, and a long string of green glass beads on a linked chain, of unknown provenance. The women on the card are fairies: the first peers out as she pinches a small clump from the ends of her hair, which is adorned with intricate jewels; the second is sleeping, her head resting on a budding green stem; the third is absorbed in her task as she stitches the blooming white froth of the wildflower known as Queen Anne's lace; the fourth and final fairy wears a gold crown and floating pink veil and is looking up as she measures arm lengths of what appears to be a thin golden ribbon. In nearly unreadable gold script against the dark-green background, the card reads: *To me the flowers are passing dear, I see them all when thou art near. / When you are near I've bliss supreme, I feel contentment glow, I wish no other joy*

to feel or happiness to know. / My hope, my heaven, my trust must be,
My gentle guide, in following thee. The mysterious green beads that
hung beside the card seemed very old to me even forty years ago.

There was a push-button lock on the doorknob I almost never
used, and the one time I remember trying it, I accidentally
locked everyone out of the bathroom on my way out. Uncle Al,
Joanna's oldest brother, was a locksmith, and he drove over in his
van filled with keys. Everyone was irritated with me. I hid in my
bedroom and cried.

❧

I CRIED EASILY. My emotional reactions were big and came
in overwhelming waves, and I often retreated to my bedroom
when I was upset. My mother didn't have a real room of her
own, but I did. It was red, like my grandmother's, with similar
rose-patterned wallpaper.

One time the family next door threw a party for their daughters, who were both close to my age, and I had been excluded
from the gathering, though other neighbourhood kids were
there, splashing away in their above-ground pool. I wailed as I
stared out my window into their backyard, my face crimson and
shining. My mother marched next door and expressed her
indignation at the cruelty of leaving me out, and then returned,
telling me that I was now invited. I was so happy, and I threw
on my pink ruffled suit, flying over there, feeling triumphant,
victorious in the face of injustice. Their father punctured my
pleasure with a false smile and the remark, "We didn't realize

you would want to come—just make sure you don't pee in the pool." I saw in the truculent expressions of the sisters that, though my mother had intervened successfully, they still clearly didn't want me there. It was as if the colour drained from everything, and I wasn't sure where I wanted to be: an obvious intruder there in the full glare of the summer sun, surrounded by the suburban chain-link fences that delineated each yard, or back in my own room, where it was cool and dark.

The items of furniture in my room were all antiques, like all the furniture in the house, inherited from dead family members or picked up for almost nothing at second-hand shops. My bed was so tall that my grandfather built me a stepping stool in his workshop so that I could climb up and pull myself under the covers. I loved the ritual of bedtime. Even if I saw little of her during the day, my mother would read to me before I fell asleep from a book of nursery rhymes and short moral fables that stressed the value of hard work. "'Now see here!' said their mother from the green garden patch, 'If you want any breakfast, you just come here and scratch!'"

On the windowpane beside the bed, a Tot Finder sticker, bright red and reflective, with the figure of a firefighter carrying the body of a small girl out of a burning house.

❦

JOANNA'S CORNER OF the basement contained two pieces of furniture: her bed and a small wooden hutch painted mint green, lined with black-and-white contact paper covered in illustrations of beautiful topless women wearing ornate arm bands, their hair styled like the women of Greek and Roman statues. These women lounged in an endlessly repeating antechamber, among roses and vines. Their bodies floated close to each other and yet each seemed lost in her own thoughts, disconnected from those floating above or below or beside her. Some wore their hair in pins, others in loose waves over their shoulders, flowing like water. Some had arms raised, while others crossed their arms modestly over their breasts. All gazed down or into the middle distance, seeming both aware and unaware of being watched. Wearing garland skirts, jewelled arm bands, ornate belts, they were ladies of prestige, powerless in their ease, resigned to the state of being offered for admiration at all times. They floated eternally behind the doors of the hutch, whose wire screens had also been painted mint green.

Inside this hutch were two pairs of glittering dancing shoes, one silver and one gold, that I never saw anyone wear. I would sit in front of the hutch and hold them in my hand. Behind me, in the centre of the room, there was a large oval table that belonged to my grandparents. This is where Joanna stacked the tips she made as a waitress at a nearby pizzeria, building dull columns of nickel and copper, short, fat towers of quarters and a thin, shining tower of dimes. She would let me help make paper rolls of these coins to take to the bank, filling the stiff tubes and folding the tough corners down on each end.

When I tired of counting coins, I would lie down on her bed, which was low to the ground and covered in something she called a memory quilt, a haphazard pattern of velvet and satin squares cut from dresses she had worn to school dances: blues, greens, lavender. I petted the surface of each block with the same care I gave to the cat, keeping my stroke in the direction that felt smoothest under my fingers. It was luxurious. Then I grabbed the deck of tarot cards by the bed, shuffled them and arranged the cards across the quilt for close study.

"People are afraid of the Death card," Joanna told me, "but it almost never means someone is going to die. It's all about rebirth, new beginnings." In the picture, a skeleton wearing a suit of armour rode his horse through a valley. His valley, I guessed. I studied the black rose emblazoned on Death's banner.

"The Tower's the one to worry about," she said.

❦

IN THE BACKYARD of my grandparents' house, the neighbours were blocked by walls of green: a compost pile behind the garage, rows of tomatoes, ruffled lettuce, long beans in the back. At the end of a short brick path stood an arbour woven with wide grape leaves, the vine's tight, coiled tendrils and purple-blue globes with a cloudy finish and filled with seeds. Root vegetables and herbs took their place down the far side of the house: carrot, onion, garlic, dill, sage. One year a pumpkin. And always flowers in beds, flowers in pots: foxglove, tiger lily, crocus, pansy, petunia, marigold, buttercup, zinnia. Lilac by the drive and roses near the herbs. In summer we ate salads with borage flowers, pale-blue stars with black hearts. I loved to climb the apple tree in the backyard. I would disappear, little empress of the ferns below, hidden within a pretend forest that reached as far as the arms of a single fruit tree, an imagined wild wood between two garages.

One fall, for an art project, Joanna made a life-sized man out of blue fabric and propped him in a folding lawn chair in the backyard, as if he were lounging in the garden. She'd dressed him in Levi's, a chambray shirt, a brown corduroy newsboy hat. His face was smooth, featureless. She had posed him carefully, with one squishy leg crossed over the other in a relaxed, masculine manner. I remember his long, flat, blue, misshapen feet. I jumped into his lap, threw my arms around his sagging neck and said, "Daddy!" And we all laughed and laughed.

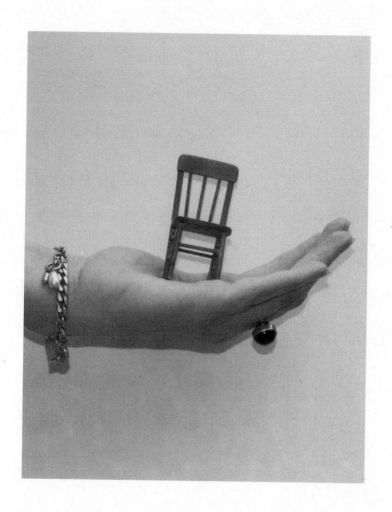

abalone / abandonment / ability / abuse
accident / acceptance / accuracy / acrobat / action
adaptivity / addiction / adjustment / admiration
admission / adolescence / adornment / adulation
adult / adultery / adventure / advocate / aesthetics
affair / affect / affection / affinity / affirmation
affliction / affordability / agate / age / agency
aggression / agitation / agony / aid / aide
airplane / album / alchemy / alcoholic / alikeness
allegation / allegiance / alleviation / alley
alliance / alligator / allocation / allowance / allure
aloneness / alphabet / alteration / alternative
amalgamation / amateur / ambience / ambiguity
ambition / ambivalence / ambush / amelioration
amendment / ammunition / amnesia
amorphousness / amulet / amusement
anachronism / analogy / anatomy / anecdote
angel / anger / anguish / animism / annihilation
annoyance / anodyne / answer / antagonist
antelope / antenna / anticipation / antidote
antique / anxiety / apparition / appendectomy
applause / apples / appointment / appropriateness
approval / archive / arduousness / argument
aria / arrangement / array / arrival / A R T
articulation / artifice / artist / ash / assembly
assent / assessment / assets / assimilation
assistance / association / Ativan / attack
attendant / attitude / attraction / aureola
author / autonomy / avoidance / awakeness
awareness

IN 1975, THE Kresge-Ford Building opened in downtown Detroit, home of what was then called the Center for Creative Studies—an art college that has tweaked its name over the years but was always referred to locally by its initials, CCS. That same year, Joanna began to take classes there. The building was of great interest to me as a child because, with its concrete columns and exaggerated joints, it looked as if it were constructed from Tinkertoys. This is what we said, my mother and I: that her art school looked like it was made out of Tinkertoys. Was she the first to see the building this way, or was I? When I look at pictures of it now, the aging beige surface looks stark, even grim, but when I was a little girl, it was clearly a space designed for play.

Every Saturday for the next four years, Joanna would drive us a half hour down Woodward Avenue to her life drawing and painting classes. I would sit with her and draw the nude models in crayon—a waxy green thicket-thick seventies bush, carefully articulated, red-polished toes. Sometimes there were games of chase or hide-and-seek with a few of the professors' and art models' kids in the hallway. I loved being there, following my mother through halls that reeked of turpentine, climbing onto paint-splattered metal stools. Joanna's professors indulged my presence. Once, memorably, one professor shared a Nestle Crunch bar with me, praising my scribbles. "You look like sisters," men would say every time we walked into a room together.

Joanna wanted to be the French-Venezuelan artist Marisol when she grew up. As a teenager, she had seen Marisol's work at the Detroit Institute of Arts in a travelling exhibit sponsored by New York's Museum of Modern Art. It was a groundbreaking show and Marisol's public image was youthful and glamorous. My fifteen-year-old mother was impressed with the work, but she was even more impressed that the work was included at all, exhibited alongside bold-name male artists of the day such as Rosenquist, Indiana and Oldenburg. Marisol's choice to use only her first name seemed subversive. Joanna thought, Oh, a woman who is an artist. An artist who is a woman. *That's what I want to be.* When she was a single mother, working part-time at a pizza parlour and living with her parents, not everyone understood her decision to study fine arts. But she told me it was something she *had* to do.

Later, I understood that Detroit's art museum had been a site of transformation for my mother. It was our church. As we walked through its halls, she would share memories of her history there, pointing out, for example, where she had her first kiss with an exchange student beneath a wrought iron circular staircase.

My mother's ambitions were ill-defined, but they were clearly real to her. She once complained about a time when my father had deeply insulted her during a fight with the accusation "You told me you were an artist!"

"As if I weren't one," she hissed, her anger still fresh.

By the mid- to late seventies, the Cass Corridor scene that my mother had skirted the edge of as a teenager—going to coffee shops where John Sinclair read poetry, getting thrown out of the Grande Ballroom for looking too young—had faded somewhat in its intensity, but several of her professors had come up during that time, and she liked brushing up against the counterculture in this comfortable way. Years later I learned she'd interviewed for some kind of job at *Creem* magazine, but the laid-back after-hours schedule turned her off. "Did you meet Lester Bangs?" I asked her eagerly, but she'd never heard of the infamous music journalist so ardently admired by all the guys who had ever made me a mixed tape. "I had a child; I couldn't work all night," she countered when I told her I couldn't believe she'd missed that opportunity.

She didn't feel any pull to a wilder lifestyle, and as far as I know, after I was born, she rarely, if ever, went out at night, unless it was on a date. Dates were dinner, maybe a movie. She didn't hang around smoky bars to see live music, she didn't attend art parties wearing outrageous outfits. I don't even remember her paying attention to the shows at local galleries. After I grew up, I was the one who was desperate to find myself in the theatre of the night, and I was fascinated with the legends of the Detroit of my mother's youth. What was it like, I asked her when she was visiting me in Toronto so many years later. From what I'd read, there had been a miniature, grittier Haight–Ashbury of disaffected dropouts who hung around Cass Avenue, near Wayne State University, CCS and the Detroit Institute of Arts. Scrappy young people living communally, espousing radical politics, making art, shaking shit up. "I went down there some-times," she said, searching her memory for specifics. "There wasn't a lot there. I remember some girls selling candles."

My mother included me in all of her pursuits, and so her pur-suits were limited to where she could include me. After class we would walk across Woodward to the art museum, which was free, and we would have something to eat in the Kresge Court cafete-ria. I remember sandwiches slowly spinning inside a cloudy glass carousel and a large brown metal box that made hot drinks when you punched the right buttons. We would insert coins into the box and dark liquid would stream into small Styrofoam cups, delivering coffee for Jo-Jo, hot chocolate for me.

We toured the remarkable permanent collection there every weekend. Early on, the two works of art I loved best from these trips to the museum were both by Claes Oldenburg: a giant three-way electrical plug made from wood that was hung over the stairs, and an ice cream bar made of a melting, bubbling alphabet. At four years old, I understood these pieces easily; they were direct sources of delight. By the time I was seven or eight, my taste grew more conservative—as Joanna later pointed out to me—and I gravitated toward the heavy religious paint-ings of earlier centuries.

❦

A FEW YEARS ago, going through my mother's emails, I found the contact information for a guy she had been friends with at CCS, a fellow student. He had sent a note to let her know about the death of one of their professors, adding, "I'm not sure if you want to get this kind of news or not." I reached out to him from my own account and explained that my mother was sick. We emailed back and forth a few times. He was excited to be in touch, telling me he thought of my mother every few months, though he hadn't seen her in decades. He agreed to share anything he could remember about my mother from their art school days and sent me several detail-rich accounts of their shared experiences.

He told me about Joanna breaking down in class one time when I wasn't with her. One of their professors had played a record with a long performance poem by John Giorno called "Eating Human Meat." The poem details the rape and torture of two ten-year-old boys at a construction site, describing the violence in graphic detail as the abusers set fire to one boy's hair and dangle the other out of the window. Joanna's large brown eyes became glassy with tears. Early in his career Giorno had worked with Bob Moog—inventor of the modern synthesizer—to create a recording system that looped lines of his poems into circular, repeating samples, so that his voice echoed in an insistent, chanting rhythm. As the poem continued to play in their classroom, Giorno's voice drove back and forth over each gruesome stage of the assault it described. By the time he reached the lines "and ripped their assholes open, and ripped their assholes open, and ripped their assholes open, and ripped their assholes open," my mother began to sob, losing control, unable to stop or calm down. Everyone else in the class tried to ignore her, embarrassed by her emotional excess. The guy she'd been friends with thought at the time that her reaction was uncool, a sign of weakness. But he wrote to me that as he'd aged, he had come to see it as evidence that she was far more empathetic than anyone else in the class.

If he could go back in time, he said, he would take her in his arms and hold her until she stopped crying, until she was okay, instead of turning away as he did.

❧

IT WAS A thrill when I had the opportunity to join the handful of other kids hanging around in the halls, as we were completely unsupervised. I was the youngest and followed their lead. One time we were chasing each other around a small exhibit of ceramic sculptures and I lost my balance, barrelling into one of the pedestals and knocking a work—one Joanna had singled out with admiration before class—to the floor, where it smashed into bits. There has been no sound as loud as that one in my life: the crash and then adults running into the hallway from every door, men yelling, my sobs, my mother's fear. I can still see the face of her professor, feel how angry he was with me.

Beyond the terror I felt over destroying this valuable object— and about getting in trouble in such a public way—an ongoing source of stress for many days afterward was whether or not my mother was going to have to pay for the lost piece. I remember watching Joanna on the phone with the artist at my grandparents' house as we all listened in. She nervously twisted the long black cord that connected the heavy receiver to the wall-mounted rotary-dial phone in the kitchen. The cord was long enough that she could have sat on a chair in the dining room, but instead she stood through the whole call, pacing the few feet the cord would allow, her voice almost too soft to hear. I knew we didn't have any money to replace the destroyed sculpture. When she hung up the phone, my mother's body went limp with relief. It had been a gift to his art practice, he'd told her. The accident had helped him confront the fragility of all artistic labour. I didn't understand this; all I knew was that I could breathe again.

Even as I grew older, I continued to shadow my mother at her classes. More and more, I no longer roamed the halls with the other stray kids but sat with my mother, studiously drawing at her side. I distinctly recall one of the last times I tagged along. At this point, Joanna had already switched from a focus on fine arts to the advertising and commercial design programme, but she loved drawing too much not to take at least one life drawing class each term. On this Saturday, when my mother and I arrived, I was shocked at the sight of the model, at the front of the class on a riser, as usual—but this time a man. Before this moment there had only been female models in the classes I'd attended. Their nudity never seemed strange to me, even though I had rarely seen my own mother naked. I had certainly never seen a naked man before. And here, at the centre of the room, was an adult penis.

By this time, I was eight years old and had cobbled together a crude image of what a penis might look like based on whispered schoolyard descriptions. I was not prepared for the existence of testicles, though, and when I saw them hanging behind the model's penis, I didn't fully understand what I was looking at. My mother looked first at the model and then at my reaction to the model— I've never had a poker face and I'm sure my horror was easy to read—and suggested I spend the class reading in the hallway.

I had brought along a science book. It wasn't for school, I just liked to look at the secrets of the universe. The book was full of colour-coordinated tables and focused captions, and soon I was lost in it and able to forget about the model. As I sat in the hallway, a woman came out to talk to me. She was kind and had genuine interest in what I was reading. I showed her the picture I was carefully studying, of the many different layers of rock below the ground we walk on. The illustration revealed what is hidden in our daily life: so many different colours of rock, varieties of hardness as one drills farther down through the evidence of time. I imagined piercing through the crust, through the mantle, down, down through the outer core and toward the inner core, arriving finally at that hot ball of light at the centre of this world, our own underground sun.

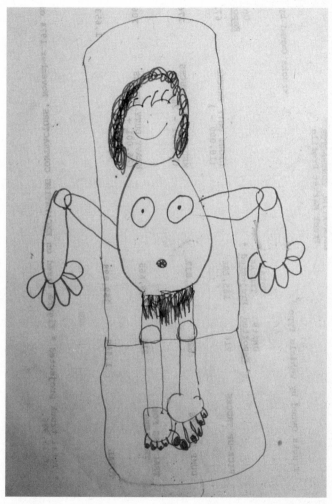

NUDE, 1978

madness / magazines / M A G I C / magnet
magnitude / maladaption / malaise / manacle
management / manatee / mandate / mandolin
manifestation / manipulation / mannerism
manuscripts / marionette / mark / marmalade
marriage / mask / mass / match / maternity
maze / mediation / medicine / meditation
medium / medulla / melancholy / melodrama
melody / membrane / memento / memoir / men
menagerie / menopause / mentality / mercilessness
mercury / mercy / mesh / messages / method
metronome / mettle / midriff / migraines / mild
milk / mime / mimeograph / mind / mine
miniature / mint / minx / mire / mirror
miscarriage / mischief / misdirection / misery
misfortune / misjudgment / misplacement / mist
mistake / mobilization / molestation / monarch
money / monkey / monsters / mood / moon / moral
mortgage / mosaic / motherhood / motivation
motorcycle / mould / mountain / mourner
movement / muck / muddle / mural / murk
murmur / muse / museum / music / mutability
muzzle / myopia / mystery / myth

MY GRANDMOTHER WAS a legend in her own house. Although she had not been conventionally beautiful, beauty mattered to her. She had style. For the first decade of my life I was my grandmother's best audience. We spent a lot of time together, me playing on the floor of the living room as she sat in her nest, a mass-market paperback copy of Marion Weinstein's *Positive Magic* or Antonia Fraser's *Mary Queen of Scots* on the table beside her. I'd make spaceships out of cardboard cups cut from egg cartons, or pore over sheets of font samples my mother brought home from her new job as a keyliner at a magazine publisher downtown. When I visited her at work, I'd watch as she carefully dragged an X-acto knife through thick glue-backed paper, as she sliced and laid out lines of text in measured columns before they were sent to camera.

"When I met your grandmother, her eyes were so dark they were black. I found her very attractive," my grandfather would say within earshot of my grandmother.

"My eyes were never black," my grandmother would correct him. "They were swamp-coloured."

Then she would recite the poem she had written about her looks. I never saw it typed up, but I've put the line breaks where I heard them.

My eyes, two swamp-coloured pools
my lips   two blood-red worms
crawling across my face.

My grandmother's eyes did have a muddy quality to them. She carried herself with a certain arch coyness still visible when I see her in photos from the 1930s through the late 1960s. She often stood with her hand on her hip, and I stood the same way by the time I was four. My grandparents never had much money, but that didn't stop my grandmother from working every bit of glamour she could. Fur-collared coats, net-veiled hats, heels, lipstick. She wore a minidress to her daughter's 1960-something wedding. (For historical context, my aunt—the bride—also wore a minidress to that same wedding.)

In the sixties, my grandmother had saved up money she made teaching high school English and got a facelift. It didn't hold up well, or perhaps it hadn't come out properly in the first place; her right eye drooped slightly in the lower lid. When I knew her, she wore thick glasses, her shoulders were bowed, her hands were covered in liver spots, her belly was round. I remember my grandmother, not usually interested in Hollywood gossip, more than once repeating a story that Vivien Leigh had lost her mind when she lost her looks. The implication was, she understood.

She would quote Shakespeare while biting her thumb—"'Do you bite your thumb at me?' 'Oh no, sir, not at you, sir. But I bite my thumb'"—and recite Dorothy Parker's "One Perfect Rose" from memory. She knew there was another life she was supposed to be living. In later life she joined the Daughters of the American Revolution and became a regent of her local chapter. She loved all the pomp, loved that no one else could start eating until she had taken "the OB"—the official bite. In a letter to my father, my mother wrote about how power suited her mother: "She always was sort of a frustrated general."

My grandmother read me *Ivanhoe* from the set of Waverley Novels that had belonged to her father, an alcoholic and charming womanizer whom she worshipped all her life. She would perform "The Elephant's Child" from Kipling's *Just So Stories* for the family, the neighbours, anyone, using different voices for each character and hamming up the elephant's part when the jaws of the crocodile were clamped securely around his nose.

After enrolling as a university freshman in her late thirties, my grandmother went on to become a high school English teacher and wrote a master's thesis on the women in Tennessee Williams's plays. She had been pursuing a Ph.D. but dropped out. I was told it was to help take care of me. She remained an autodidact, always had books beside her. Equally fascinated with the Shakers, bomb-shelter-stocking survivalists and legends of the wise women of pre-Christian villages in Europe, she sat in her nest, reading, and I sat beside her, listening. She talked to me as if I was her peer.

WE WERE MEMBERS of the YMCA, and my grandmother would take me there sometimes when she went to do laps in the pool. We would drive there in her pale-blue Pontiac LeMans, and she would change into her old-lady swimsuit, the kind with a skirt and bloomers. She topped this off with a plastic swim cap—but not the kind with flowers all over it like some of the other ladies; she wasn't that whimsical—and goggles. Then she would swim the breaststroke. She seemed very, very old to me in this act of working hard to stay as young as possible. And she did work hard: she had once given herself a hernia by doing thousands of sit-ups, trying to flatten her stomach, which had been rounded by tumours.

My grandmother had undergone a radical hysterectomy a decade before I was born. The doctors were doing exploratory surgery, and while she was still under anaesthetic, they asked my grandfather for permission to remove her uterus. "I didn't know what else to do. A doctor tells you that it needs to be done . . ." he said to me once, after she'd died, tears in his eyes. She woke up to the news that her uterus was gone.

Years later, bone cancer ate her hip away. She was in pain for a long time, but it took a while before we knew what was wrong. I remember her being miserable when the family gathered to celebrate my grandparents' fiftieth wedding anniversary; she glowered and scowled in the corner. My mother said that my grandmother was dependent on my grandfather for practical things—he did the gardening and dealt with the finances—but that my grandfather was dependent on her emotionally. It was a drag for her when he retired and spent his time hanging around the house in shabby clothes. She liked to see a man in a tie, walking out the door.

All through my childhood, my grandmother told me ghost stories. She would recount in gripping detail how she had heard a voice calling her while she played the piano in the 1940s. She had started walking toward the basement, where the voice seemed to be, until she remembered she was alone in the house. The next day she received a telegram saying that her beloved brother—who described himself to his friends as "five foot four inches of pure hell"—had died in battle on the Italian front. She would also tell me that when her sister had died in Montana, my grandmother's watch stopped on her wrist in Michigan.

She promised me that if she could return as a ghost after she died, she would come visit me. But though she has shown up in many of my dreams, I have yet to see her walking around the house.

I remember a documentary we watched together when I was in fourth grade. I think it aired on PBS—she loved PBS and Reagan—and it was about the history of witchcraft in Europe. It was a corrective bit of propaganda, framed by 1970s resistance to official accounts. What appealed to my grandmother was the image of an older woman who was powerful rather than invisible. The "wise woman" owned property, owned her own life. Most importantly, she owned knowledge and skill that the community depended on. She oversaw the twin gates of childbirth and death. (Sometimes those two gates swung open in the same room.) Her value increased rather than decreased as she aged; her experience was honoured and respected. My grandmother dreamed of such a world, in which she might be a true matriarch.

❧

I WOULD SPEND hours looking at ads for giant dolls in my grandmother's reproduction Sears, Roebuck catalogue from the 1920s. I wanted the biggest doll, the most extravagant doll, the one with brown hair like mine. In 1929 she cost $3.99. My grandmother knew I pined for this impossible doll, and so she wrote me a spell that would enable me to reach through time and drag this doll into the present. The spell involved placing a branch in a jar and setting it in the centre of a circle to signify the sacred universal tree. It also required me to perform a solitary ceremony every night for a full week. I soon gave up and left the spell unfinished. Part of me found it to be more labour than I was motivated to perform, but the other part of me was afraid. I was afraid that it might not work, and then my belief in magic would be challenged. Better not to try.

My grandmother liked the idea that I wanted this antiquated doll, illustrated only by a small line drawing and a few lines of descriptive copy. She didn't approve of the "vulgar" dolls advertised on television, the rubbery ones reeking of baby powder, the unthinkable ones that ate and shat fake food into fake diapers. And though I never held the old doll in my hands, I've never forgotten it in all these years, and perhaps that is a kind of magic of its own.

gaff / game / gamine / gap / garden / gate
gauze / geckos / gemstones / genetics / gentility
geranium / ghost / gift / giggles / gingham
giraffe / glass / globe / glory / gloss / glow / glyph
gnome / goddess / gold / goner / goodness / goof
gorilla / gossip / gouache / grace / gradient
grandparents / grapefruit / graphics / graphite
grass / gratification / gratitude / gravestone
greed / greeting / grief / grift / groove / growth
guest / guile / guilt / G U I T A R */ guys*

I WAS EIGHT years old when my ideas of death and other dangers took on clear shape. That was the year my great-grandmother Ivy died. It was the year John Lennon was shot. And it was the year my mother and I moved out of my grandparents' home. We didn't move far—just across the street and one house to the right. Still, this was a big move for us. I continued to spend lots of time with my grandparents, but now my mother began to experiment with her own domestic projects and I was her helper, her partner. We ate our first meal in our new home together on a second-hand bistro set in the dining room, which was also the laundry room. The dish was something my mother called tomato rarebit (I heard "rabbit"), a kind of tomato paste on toast. Living on our own was an adventure, I thought, like camping in the backyard.

This was the first time my mother had ever rented her own place, a place with her name on the lease. She hung her paintings on the walls and placed tall red glass votive candles on the mantel over the fireplace. A fireplace! How eccentric that house was, with its red shag carpet, accordion doors and faux wood walls. It had been owned by a bachelor, who had married and moved into a bigger house. All the other houses on the block were filled with young families or old people. None were very big, but this one was very, very small: barely two bedrooms, no basement. Its tiny footprint made for a deep backyard on the standard-size lot.

We brought over from Grandma's house our antique beds and a few uncomfortable chairs and my mother's steamer trunk. The one new thing my mother bought for herself was a guitar—a nylon-string classical acoustic guitar, which she chose because nylon would be much easier on the pads of her fingers than steel strings. It was made from glossy blond wood and had a delicate design of mother-of-pearl in a ring around the sound hole, the mouth of the guitar. She kept it in a black hardcase lined with thick blue fur that I loved to pet; it reminded me of the fur on my hand puppet of Grover from *Sesame Street*.

My mother found a guitar teacher and paid for enough lessons to learn the chords necessary to play anything in *The Beatles Songbook*, a thick collection that we left open between us as we sang. One of my favourites was "Across the Universe," a song that first appeared in 1969 as part of a compilation called *No One's Gonna Change Our World*, with the tagline "The Stars Sing for the World Wildlife Fund." It ended up on the Beatles' last record, *Let It Be*, which we didn't own. Singing this song, I was struck by the image of words streaming out of a paper cup, like water, like rain. "Nothing's going to change my world," we sang again and again, lost in the pleasure of repetition, our voices reaching toward Lennon's insistence on permanence even as our world changed faster than we could see.

❦

THIS WAS THE year my mother threw her first and only party. Our small house was filled with people. Who were they? Friends from work, friends from art school. I lay in my dark bedroom and listened to the hum of the conversations. After I'd gone to the bathroom, I had left the door of my bedroom ajar on purpose so I could hear more clearly: people talking, laughing and dancing to music, all outside my door. My door, which wasn't solid but hinged in the middle and made of slatted wood that let in thin strips of light even when it was closed tight. I was wearing footed pyjamas that were already a little too small, the zipper stretched along the short crotch, a small hole where the fuzzed fabric met the thin, plasticky pad of the foot. I worried the hole with my big toe as I lay in the semi-dark.

At some point a guy floated into my room, all smiles and jovial inquiry. What did I think of this activity in my house? He sat at the edge of my bed, his push-broom moustache seeming to move around his face as he joked with me. Then he leaned forward and in a more serious tone asked me the name of my bear.

"Bow Bow," I told him.

"I can tell this is a very special bear," he said to me, picking up the stuffed toy tenderly and cradling it in his hands for a moment before tucking it back under the covers beside me. I found the man amusing. He didn't know anything about my bear.

My mother saw my door was open. My room was so small, there was only enough space for the bed and the dresser and a short lane of carpet between them. The drawers of my dresser touched the edge of the bed when I opened them. There was only enough space for my mother to stand just inside the door frame, left hand on her hip.

She said my name sharply, or the man's name, or some kind of exasperated sound that meant, *What the hell, man?* The man, I recognize in retrospect, was drunk. I could tell he was in trouble, but I thought he was nice. He laughed loosely and explained, "She was just telling me about Bow Bow."

This answer didn't satisfy my mother. Through the open door, yellow light bounced off the kitchen's linoleum floor onto her straight dark hair, her large dark eyes. Even though she was silent, her face sent out waves that reached me like a high pitch. Then she spoke.

"She has to go to sleep. "It's after her bedtime," my mother said, glaring at the guy.

He shrugged and laughed again. "What? Okay, okay," he said. He stood up, shaking his head and smiling, holding his hands in the air, his palms facing forward, like the robber in a movie who walks out of a bank knowing the cops have the place surrounded. He called good night to me over his shoulder as my mother closed the door with a snap behind her.

In the morning, I found litres of unfinished pop around the house. It was better than Halloween, and I drank nothing but Coke and Tab and Squirt for days.

Soda was a rare treat, something my grandmother would never allow in her house and that my mother wouldn't normally waste money on. We called it pop, as in "Can I have *a* pop?" for a can or "Can I have *some* pop?" for a glass. You'd buy it at the "party store," and when I was eight, I was obsessed with the junk food you could buy at a party store.

There was one such store called Shindig down the street from my cousin Ann's house. Ann was my Uncle Al's youngest daughter, born only a few months after me. Around the time my mother and I moved into our first house, I started to spend the occasional night at Ann's house, which was about a mile away from us. At Ann's house I could pour myself a giant glass of 7 Up like it was no big deal; I didn't even have to ask. We'd walk down to Shindig and buy Hubba Bubba, Bubblicious, Bubble Yum—we especially loved the fancy new kinds of gum that came in fat squares with a syrupy liquid-sugar core that would ooze out through your teeth when you bit down. Food and schedules were heavily policed at home, but it was a free-for-all at Ann's house. We were left alone to watch TV, and no one told us we had to brush our teeth or go to bed.

❦

THE DAY JOHN LENNON was shot, Joanna retreated into her bedroom and shut the door. I stood outside and listened to her listening to the clock radio by her bed. I heard the DJ asking for a minute of silence. My mother too was asking for a minute of silence. My mother was alone in her room on the bed in the dark, and I stood outside the door . . . and I couldn't stand it. I didn't know why, but I couldn't stand it.

"Mom?" I called out. She was silent. "Mom?" I called again. Silence. "Mom?"

"What?" she said. Through the door and through her teeth. I needed to come in. I needed to be on the right side of the door.

❧

I HAD A hazy idea of death. When my great-grandmother Ivy died, my mother explained death by reading to me from *The Little Prince* by Saint-Exupéry. She read the part where the benevolent alien prince reveals his plans to his kind but not always comprehending friend, the aviator. The Little Prince explains to the aviator that he's made an arrangement with the snake, the snake in the desert that the aviator fears. This snake, the Little Prince says, is going to help him go home, to his own planet, where his vain, vulnerable, beautiful rose waits for him to return. Don't follow me when I go see the snake, he says. It will look as if I'm in pain. It will look as if I'm dying. Don't come. But of course, the aviator doesn't listen, and the aviator watches the Little Prince die, and the aviator grieves the loss of his friend, and the aviator blames the snake.

I was taking a bath when my mother sat on the floor of the bathroom and read this to me. It was a book she had read to me many times, but never only this scene. She was crying.

"Great-grandma Ivy died, didn't she?" I asked my mother before she could tell me. My mother nodded, tears streaming down her face, and I glowed with pride that I'd figured it out. I'd connected the dots. I'd solved the puzzle.

Ivy was Grandma's mother. She lived in Montana, in a trailer surrounded by roses, right by Rock Creek, where her father had bought land from members of the Crow Nation at the end of the nineteenth century. Ivy had visited us a couple of years before she died. In a photo from that trip, I sit in her lap. Ivy is wearing a polyester pantsuit in coral and a matching coral-and-white polka-dot shirt with giant pointing lapels. Her hair is silver and she wears it in short, tight curls. I wear a denim jumper my grandmother made me with a light-blue gingham shirt layered lumpily underneath.

What I knew about the arc of Ivy's life was that she had travelled by covered wagon as an infant and had lived to see a man on the moon. She had married three times and taught herself Spanish, and at the age of eighty she had climbed into a doorless cargo plane so she could see some important ruins in Mexico. I was sad she had died, but as I watched my mother from the tub, what I felt most was the joy I still experience when I think I've cracked open the true and dazzling meaning of any story.

❦

MY MOTHER WAS the youngest of four kids—two boys and two girls. My mother's sister and the younger of her brothers had both moved away, raising their own kids in the south, Texas and Florida respectively. Like my mother, her other brother still lived in the same suburb where they grew up.

My cousin Ann lived with her older brother and sister and her mother and father in a single-floor two-bedroom house covered in powder-blue aluminum siding with a cement porch and black railings. The living room furniture was covered in soft brown velour, stained in many places, and the TV was hooked up to both VHS and Betamax units. It was in Ann's house that I met the world of contemporary culture. We watched *Grease* over and over, Olivia Newton-John transforming into a shimmying greaser's girl in her off-the-shoulder leotard. We stayed up as late as we wanted, watching Bowzer line-dance in Converse sneakers and a ten-gallon hat on Barbara Mandrell's country music variety show. Sometimes we managed to stay awake for at least the beginning of *Saturday Night Live*. We watched *The Blue Lagoon*, and I understood it to be scandalous—teenagers swimming naked through the deep waters of paradise.

It was around this time that my uncle started saying I looked like Brooke Shields, the fourteen-year-old star of the film, though nobody my own age seemed to think so. When I was six, I'd seen Brooke Shields on the cover of a *Seventeen* magazine that had been left on the picnic table at the Tot Lot one day. Her face haunted me, although I couldn't say why; I only knew that she looked like a child and an adult at the same time. Now I would say I intuited that she was trapped at the crossroads between two contradictory states of being: innocence and experience. The effect was mesmerizing and a little scary. I couldn't read her expression; she faced the camera with confidence, and yet I saw the ripple of a tug-of-war between defiance and fear in her green eyes, in the set of her mouth and jaw. She looked as if she had seen something I hadn't yet seen. She looked vulnerable and resilient. She was an ocean away from me. She was thirteen. She was practically a grown-up.

I liked that my uncle thought I looked like her.

At Ann's, we were left alone for the most part, though sometimes I would quietly study her father's tattoos as he smoked and played a hand-held electronic chess game at the dining room table. He could sometimes beat the computer. My mother said he was very smart, that no one realized how smart he was. He was the only person I'd ever seen with tattoos. I'd heard my mother and my grandparents refer to the fact that he had gotten them overseas when he was in the navy. He had a large dragon on one arm and a panther on the other; the outlines of the indigo designs were already starting to blur a little. On each hand he had small anchors over his knuckles, which he hated and had tried to burn off with the salicylic acid they sell to treat warts. He was shy with me and kept to himself when I was around.

❦

ONE NIGHT, ANN and I were in the living room playing Barbies. I was fitting a small yellow high-heeled mule onto the plastic blonde's over-arched foot when my mother came to the door. She had come to pick me up, she said, even though I was supposed to be spending the night. It was late, past my bedtime at home. I didn't understand what was happening and my mother didn't explain. She wouldn't come in, just stood outside the front screen door and told me I needed to get my things and go, while my uncle laughed and tried to talk to her. Later, I figured out that he had been drunk, though I hadn't been aware of it. All night he had been at the outer edges of my attention. Joanna was angry, but she didn't yell. No negotiation, just firm instruction. "Damian, we're leaving. Say good night to Ann," she said.

She had called her brother on the phone, or he had called her, and—had they fought? Had he said something disturbing? Or was it just his slurring voice that made her get in the car and pull me out of the house that night? She never told me.

My mother almost never drank. Allan was eleven years older than her, and he started drinking when he was a teenager, so she had watched him drink her whole life. There had been at least one short spell of sobriety, but it hadn't lasted. "When he told me he didn't need AA anymore, I knew he'd start drinking again," she told me once.

My mother had never been drawn to alcohol or other drugs. She had no tolerance for either and no real interest in that particular brand of escape. Our nights at home were quiet. Before we could afford a television, and for years afterward, my mother and I spent hours with the guitar between us. On weekends sometimes we would go to the music store to pick out sheet music for songs such as Jackson Browne's "Tender Is the Night," Juice Newton's "Queen of Hearts" and Linda Ronstadt's "Blue Bayou," along with old hits made famous by the Shirelles and the Supremes. We bought sheet music instead of buying records. We sat on the floor of the living room and sang love songs that were shadowed by doubt—"Will you still love me tomorrow?"— love songs about connections that were tenuous and built to break, or already lost—"I'm so lonesome all the time / Since I left my baby behind"—love songs that weren't love songs at all—"Looking for somebody / Somewhere in the night." We had pleasant but not powerful voices; we shut our eyes in concentration when we strained toward notes almost out of reach. It was important to us to sound good, to sound pretty, even if we were the only ones listening. And it was always just us. My mother was too shy to sing in front of anyone else, and so I was her audience, though I spent more time wondering if my voice was good than I spent listening to her. I wanted to sing as well as she did. I wanted to sing better.

On our own, we grew closer and I studied her carefully. We were a team now. At Farmer Jack or Kroger, I'd steer her toward better deals on chocolate and butterscotch puddings for my bagged lunches. I had chores for the first time, and did my small part to keep the house clean. It seemed to me that my job was to toughen up. When we sang duets, I sang the guy's part, and our voices blended in every chorus—we never mastered harmonies—as we crooned sweet, melodic promises and the irresistible, lilting call to "stay with me stay."

> *I need you to love me*
> *I need you to day*
> *Give to me your leath er*
> *Take from me my lace*

dahlia / daisy / damage / dampness / dandelion
danger / darling / D A T E S / daughter / day
daze / dearth / death / debacle / debilitation
debt / decades / decay / deception / decline
decoupage / definition / degeneration / deletion
delicacy / delusion / dementia / denial
dependency / depletion / depression / depths
descent / designer / desire / despair / desperation
despondency / development / devolution
devotion / diagnosis / dignity / dilemma / din
dinner / disarrange / discord / disease
disengagement / disinhibition / disloyalty
disorganization / dispiritedness / dissociation
distance / distortion / distress / dive / division
divorce / doctors / dollhouse / door / dopamine
dotage / double / doubt / dragon / drain
drawer / drawing / dream / dresser / drummer
drunk / dulcimer / duress / dyad / dysfunction

INSTEAD OF A couch for our living room, my mother had bought a wicker loveseat at Pier 1 and spray-painted it white. She then covered that hard mass of poking sticks with cushions she'd made out of a thick, scratchy green fabric, along with a few matching accent pillows on which she'd sewn silky botanical-print panels. The floor was more comfortable. Backs propped against the loveseat, we'd paint our nails and watch dashing men fight bad guys on TV. Magnum, PI, prowled paradise with his moustache, Hawaiian shirt and Detroit Tigers hat, and Michael Knight hit the streets in his talking car named KITT. I studied the imperfections of our feet as the polish dried, disgusted by the length and shape of my own toes. Sometimes we would soak our feet and scrub them with a pumice stone. Together, we read the "Private Time" column in *Glamour* magazine, devotees of their recommendations of hot baths, journalling and creative visualization.

My mother still worked as a keyliner, but she dreamed of breaking into advertising, though she hadn't been able to convince the woman running a local Women in Advertising club to let her attend their networking events. After watching the movie *Return of the Jedi*, we also aspired to the kind of mind control practised by superheroes in space. To make her feel better, I made my mother a drawing in which she was the cover star of an industry mag, with a headline celebrating her as the "First Jedi Ad-Knight," her billowing cape lined with pockets holding pencils, X-acto knives and rulers.

We had moved again, out of the small house across the street from my grandparents' house and into a small townhouse apartment a couple of miles away, in a neighbouring suburb. Now that we were out of my grandmother's immediate sight-lines, my mother's dating life became much more visible to me. It seemed to me that she was always dating; sometimes there would be a steady boyfriend for a little while, but never for very long. Often, she would be dating more than one guy at a time. This didn't seem strange to me. Years later, although the faces of the men on TV remain clear to me, the faces of my mother's dates are blurred. Even at the time, my mother and I called one particular pair Turkey-Face One and Turkey-Face Two—they both had ginger-haired beards, but their faces were interchangeable to me.

Sometimes, maybe to save on a sitter, she would entertain her date at home. She had bought a ten-dollar hibachi grill the size of a dinner plate and she would cook skewered meat and vegetables over it on our back stoop, which itself was barely larger than the grill. On one special occasion she prepared lobster tails, which I dunked into a small dish of lemon butter upstairs in my bedroom. I was happy to be upstairs that night, because we had borrowed my grandparents' small black-and-white television and I was allowed to watch the Charlie Brown Valentine's Day episode while I ate. On other occasions I would listen to top-ten countdowns on my clock radio. If I managed to stay awake late enough, I could hear local Detroit DJ the Electrifying Mojo play Eddy Grant—"Working so hard like a soldier / Can't afford a thing on TV." After I was supposed to be asleep, I would creep down the stairs, hidden from view, and listen to my mother and these men moan as they made out in the living room, sometimes risking a peek over the banister. They were always still clothed, mashed up together on that undersized loveseat.

My mother never let her dates sleep over, and with me she maintained an appearance of innocence around her affairs. She told me she'd stopped seeing one guy because he got too handsy. "Every time we say good night, he turns into an octopus!" she exclaimed, and I nodded wisely.

It was important to my mother that I didn't know she had never been married to my father. There was one girl in my second-grade class whose parents were divorced, but she saw her father on weekends, and I knew her situation wasn't the same as mine. At school, I always left the space for *Father* blank on the forms we had to fill in every fall. In fifth grade a teacher finally asked me, "Why didn't you fill out the section for your father?"

My desk, across from one of the five Jennifers, was set up so that my back was toward the teacher's desk. I watched drifting particles of dust sparkle as they sifted toward the floor. I shrugged. "Because I don't have one," I said with a cheerful, almost swaggering note in my voice. Though I too wanted to know more about that blank space, this was the truth. That blank space was the only story I had.

From what I can tell, this is when my mother and father began to correspond. In her earliest letters to him that I found in the box he gave me, she provides bits of news about our life, along with promises that my school photos don't do me justice ("she really is quite pretty"). In one letter she thanked him for a cheque he'd sent around the holidays, which she explained she'd used to buy me a "much needed" winter coat. And then her words changed tone.

> *I am sorry to say I don't want you to come see her, I know that is probably hard for you. I hope you don't feel I'm being vindictive, but she does not know she is illegitimate, and I have no desire to break that to her at this age. When she is much older maybe I will. You have to realize that even though the money is appreciated and used, there were many years when there was none. I struggled very hard for a very long time, for a long time we had to live with my folks (over)*

The letter continues on the other side.

> *It was hard in many, many ways. And now though I appreciate the money—*

The sentence breaks off there, unfinished, and there is a squiggle on the page, as if she wasn't sure what to write next. I imagine her stopping there for some time before finishing the letter. She'd been writing with a pencil, and this section is ghostly faint, almost impossible to read, as if her hand were pulling away from the page even as she continued to write. As if she were sketching the words as lightly as possible before committing to them.

I have struggled hard to raise a child, a good child, a child that will be able to hold her own against the world some day, I won't risk what I have worked so hard to obtain. She knows the money comes from her father, but she doesn't know she's illegitimate. That's too big a thing to set on the shoulders of a child, and I won't do it. If you had always given money and come to see her I would have dealt with it, but not now, she keeps the pictures of your children in her wallet, she looks a little like Lucy. thank you, j.

I'm struck by my mother's idiosyncratic choice of punctuation in that long last line. Not even a period in between the finality of "but not now" and the news that I carried photos of his kids around with me, and the fact that I resembled his younger sister, Lucy. Reading the letter now, I'm taken by the rushing waters of that final jumbled sentence, the odd, off-rhythm pulse of it. I can feel her breathless anger and anxiety there, and also her determination to protect me. Her determination to protect me from her own sense of shame. But the shame isn't limited to her own body, it's embedded in my very existence. The shame of her failed marriage, the shame of placing her hopes and dreams in the wrong next man, the shame of acting outside the lines of family and law. The word *illegitimate*—a word I have never heard used to describe a child in my adult life, except when reading or watching historical dramas about bastard kings— described not my mother's relationships, but me. The burden my mother wanted to spare me wasn't the specific facts of my parentage, but her own shame that I had not been embraced and treasured by my father. That I hadn't been recognized. That I was not legitimate.

But I was good. A good child.

What happened between the day she wrote this letter and the day, not so many months later, that she sat me down to tell me that my father wasn't the man named on my birth certificate but another man I had never met? What changed her mind, made her think it was time for me to know this fact that had been hidden for the first ten years of my life? I don't know what made her choose the top of the stairs in our apartment as the site of this revelation. We never before or after sat together at the top of those stairs. It felt planned—maybe not the exact moment, but certainly her speech about why she had lied (to protect me from the judgment of others). When she told me, I thought about the man in my mother's high school yearbooks, the one whose name was on my birth certificate, the one I'd thought was my father.

Before our talk on the stairs, I would sometimes pull my mother's two high school yearbooks off the shelf when I was alone in the apartment to look at the man I had thought was my father. Though her yearbooks were then fewer than fifteen years old, to me they seemed like ancient artifacts. I'd study the photos of my mother with her shoulder-length flip and straight-across bangs—the same as every other girl in those black-and-white rows. And I'd check out her ex, the one she'd followed to California, the one who, it turned out, had nothing to do with me, though I continued to carry his last name around with me until I turned twenty-one, went to the courthouse and changed it to my grandmother's maiden name.

My mother cried when she told me the truth about my father. And I cried because she was crying, my eyes fixed on the multicoloured runner she had created by sewing together a long line of rag rugs that were intended to be used as doormats.

Long, lumpish strips of black-and-lilac, white-and-red, green-and-blue polyester scraps. I cried, but I didn't feel sad. Not exactly.

For years, I continued to look at photos of my mother's ex-husband and wonder what it might have been like if he'd really been my father. Would my eyes be a brighter blue? Would I be taller? It was a long time before it occurred to me that I wouldn't be me at all.

pain / painting / pair / palace / palette / panic
panther / papier-mâché / paradox / parallels
paranoia / parasites / parataxis / pardon
parent / parenthesis / parrot / partner / party
passenger / passion / passivity / password / past
patience / patient / pattern / penicillin
perception / performance / peril / permanence
permeability / perpetrator / persistence
personality / persuasiveness / pervasiveness
petulance / petunia / phobia / phoenix / phone
photo / piano / pillager / pillowcase / pills / pilot
pinworms / place / plane / play / P O E T R Y
poison / police / porousness / poverty / prayers
preciousness / prediction / premonition
prescience / prescription / presence / present
presentation / pressure / pretender / privacy
process / progression / promise / prophecy
protection / psychiatrist / psychosis / puncture
puppet / puzzle

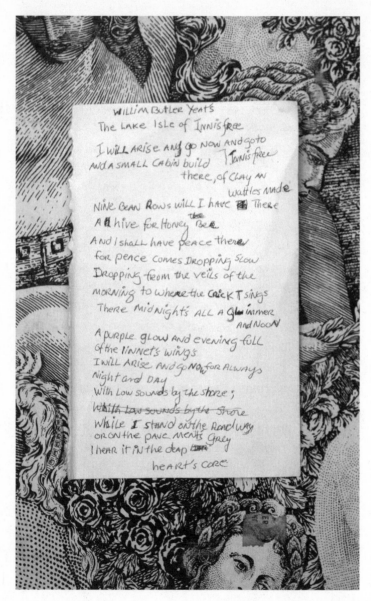

JOANNA'S SKETCHBOOK, 2012

THE CHRISTMAS I entered puberty, Joanna gave me a folder of her favourite poems and lyrics. She had used the Xerox machine at work to photocopy her selections from an anthology called *Beowulf to Beatles*, which included songwriters such as Buffy Sainte-Marie and Joni Mitchell, along with canonical poems by William Butler Yeats, Dylan Thomas and William Shakespeare. She collected about twenty or so poems in a simple purple cardstock folder that she had picked up at Perry Drugs on Coolidge. She also gave me a silver paint pen from the art store, and with this I drew a wonky wineglass on the cover. Then, in looping script above the wineglass, I wrote: *To Love, To Laughter, To Life*. This dedication made me cringe a few short years later, but it had felt like a solemn oath when I set it down.

This was a time of roller-skating parties and sticker collections. A time of unicorns, hearts and rainbows, and unicorns riding rainbows, and hearts made of rainbows, and hearts streaming through the rainbow manes of unicorns. Into this kaleidoscopic candy-coloured cream-puff daydream, my mother had inserted the words of William Butler Yeats, Emily Dickinson and Haki R. Madhubuti (who was credited in the anthology as Don L. Lee). I studied the poems with a passionate focus that I never brought to my schoolwork. I read the lyrics to Leonard Cohen's "Suzanne" so many times that I soon had it committed to memory.

My mother had been my most consistent friend before I met Andrea. We were on the local YMCA swim team, the Piranhas, together. Andrea and I watched *Xanadu* on repeat and made up erotic stories about the members of Duran Duran, writing them in a spiral notebook we passed back and forth. In these stories we were muses, just like Olivia Newton-John. For our alter egos, we looked up the names of the nine Greek muses in *The Women's Encyclopedia of Myths and Symbols*. I wanted to be the muse of lyric or love poetry, but the names sucked: Euterpe and Erato? No, thank you; I was already dealing with Damian. I wanted a pretty name, so I went with Calliope, who was the muse of epic poetry. Of course, I didn't really know what "epic poetry" was, but it sounded close enough to my ideal. Andrea wanted to be the muse of dance, but Terpsichore was also a hard sell—we didn't even know how to pronounce it. She went with Clio, the muse of history. Andrea said she liked history just fine.

❦

MEANWHILE, I WAS trying to improve my appearance. My mother had semi-successfully traded in her seventies bohemian uniform of paint-splattered Levi's and handmade ribbon-covered camisoles for an ersatz eighties power suit and perm. She still wore jeans on the weekends, or her baby-blue corduroy cut-offs with the pink calico heart patch sewed on the ass, and I thought this was when she looked the most like herself. Though she was keenly aware of how to dress for the male gaze, she never counselled me on how to be more appealing to the boys at school. From the time I was ten years old, I had day-dreamed of winning a magazine makeover that would change my life. But it was Andrea, with her sense of contemporary style, who ended up being the one to guide me a little.

One day, as we were experimenting with our outfits at her house—working with her closet—I wrapped a couple of feet of chain around my wrist as a bracelet. Andrea had recently cut her hair short and now she styled it as spiky as she could with Dippity-do, a gloopy hair gel with a consistency somewhere between rubber cement and Jell-O that came in a transparent plastic tub showing off its glorious green goo whipped through with air bubbles. It boasted the strongest hold available, in advertisements that featured the top of an androgynous head, hair standing improbably on end. Andrea's hair wasn't defying gravity as impressively as promised, but it had a stiff, hard sheen to it. You could see where the comb had travelled. I was, as usual, wearing her clothes. We put on heavy eyeliner and scowled into the mirror. Then we walked to Northwood Shopping Mall to buy gum. A stylish middle-aged Black woman in line at the drugstore when we came peeling in looked at my outfit and complimented me on my look. It was the first positive notice of what I was wearing that I had ever received from anyone outside my immediate family. It was my first positive experience with a gesture toward glamour, toward the costume of adulthood or, even better, cool teenagers. This stranger's approval was more valuable even than a boy calling me cute.

In addition to my allowance, I started to earn money by babysitting for one dollar an hour. Who were the people who put their babies in my child hands? The family next door to my grandparents were my first regular clients. The mother was young—she'd had her first of two kids at nineteen—and bought a lot of her clothes from the Spiegel catalogue. When I went to see Orchestral Manoeuvres in the Dark (OMD; *Pretty in Pink*) open up for Thompson Twins, she let me borrow her floral-print "tapestry denim" skirt suit. I had my first kiss that night from Andrea's crush, the son of a local news anchor, who made out with me sloppily as we sat in our arena seats. What I remember most is the sensation of his saliva drying on my chin, and how I surreptitiously scraped it off with my nails when no one was looking. Andrea had also recommended me to babysitting clients of hers who were heavy drinkers. One evening, the mother showed me how she'd filled an empty hairspray bottle with vodka so she could smuggle it into the place they were headed, complaining that she could still taste the chemical residue from the White Rain she'd poured down the sink. She also told me I looked like her friend, pulling out a photo of a backlit brunette in a low-cut silver lamé dress. "This is what you're going to look like when you're older, and don't be coming around my house when you do," she said.

I relied on others, like the woman at the drugstore and this boozy mom, to tell me what my face looked like, what my face might one day look like. At home, by myself, I had no face. At home, by myself, I whispered the poems "Hope Is the Thing with Feathers" and "The Lake Isle of Innisfree" to myself and heard birds and bees buzzing inside my ear.

As Dickinson's and Yeats's rhythms rattled around in my head, Andrea and I drank sparkling apple cider and watched Madonna hump the stage in layers of white lace in front of a giant fake wedding cake on MTV. We danced in wet bathing suits to Dead or Alive in front of a neighbour of Andrea's we weren't really interested in but who was close enough to our age that we still wanted to impress him. By this time I understood that what it meant to be in a bathing suit in public had changed. Instead of the high-necked navy suits we wore for our swim meets, we wore bikinis. Mine was pink and had a round plastic ring between the bunchy breast panels—even though I had no breasts beneath them. Dressed like this, we jumped around the sprinkler in Andrea's front yard, and we waved to the guy across the street, screeching his name. He looked at us for a beat, then turned around and walked back into his house.

That year I gave an oral report in my English class on the poetry of Lawrence Ferlinghetti, whose work was in the folder my mother had given me. The teacher was uncomfortable with some of the material, such as "I have not lain with Beauty all my life," but I was a believer. In a documentary about Lawrence Ferlinghetti, fellow west coast poet Michael McClure says of his work, "He's turned on two generations of young people to poetry and they've gone on from his work to reading others."

I often wonder what might have been different—how I might have been different—if these poems had not been braided into my adolescence. They articulate a white space in my mind, a room for what was missing, a place I could live inside. I didn't show these poems to anyone; they were mine. Although my mother had shared them with me, I had made them my own. She had passed them along, a gift. They gave me a private parcel of language and images that offered a bridge out of childhood. While Andrea picked up dirty ideas from older kids and R-rated movies like *Porky's*, and my classmates were reading trashy paperbacks like *Flowers in the Attic* or *Swamp Girl*, I wanted transcendence. I was interested in Ferlinghetti describing a "hungry scene" with "Beauty in my bed." I read the lyrics to Bob Dylan's seduction song "Lay Lady Lay"—which was in the folder—as a personal promise: when the time came, a guy would arrive to show me all the colours in my mind, and he would make them shine. All my rainbows, all my hearts. I wanted to be the Beauty in the bed, but I also wanted to be the man singing to win her love.

Though I had none of her vulnerable self-assurance in the face of a camera lens, I had finally reached the same age as Brooke Shields in that photo on the cover of *Seventeen*. I was somewhere in the weedy field that stretched between childhood and what lay on the other side of it. I too had made it to thirteen.

In a card to my father, thanking him for a cheque he'd sent at the end of that year, my mother wrote:

She's as big as me now. Help.

vacancy / vacation / vacillation / vacuum
valediction / valentine / valerian / validation
valley / value / vamp / van / vandal / vanity
vapour / variable / varnish / vault / vehemence
vehicle / veil / velocity / velvet / veneer
veneration / venom / ventilation / venture
veracity / verbs / verge / verification / vermilion
vermin / vernacular / versatility / version
vertigo / verve / vestige / veteran / vexation
vial / vibration / vice / vicinity / victim / victor
view / vigil / vignette / vigour / villain
villanelle / vindication / vindictiveness
vine / vinegar / violation / violence / violet
viper / virginity / virtue / visage
vision / *V I S I T A T I O N* / vitals
vivaciousness / vivisection / vixen / vocable
vocabulary / vocation / vodka / voice / void
volatility / volcano / voltage / volunteer / vomit
vortex / vow / vowel / voyage / vulgarity
vulnerability / vulture

MY MOTHER OFTEN told me a story about the time she lived in California. In this story, she began to sense an invisible presence around her. I imagine that it was especially strong when she was alone. She described the experience as feeling as if there were wings moving close to her face. She said she had felt sorry for this presence. Maybe it didn't have anywhere to go. Maybe it was lost. She first told me this story when I was quite young and repeated it more than once. Now I wonder for how long she felt this presence by her face. Was it a span of days, weeks, months? She said she felt great empathy for this presence. It had become a companion. One day she tried to communicate to the presence that, if it had nowhere to go, she would make room inside her body for it. They could share that space and stay together. *And then*, she told me, *I got pregnant with you.*

WHEN I WAS thirteen, my parents arranged a face-to-face meeting between my father and me.

I was an awkward kid and not comfortable in my body. In elementary school, I sometimes skipped recess to stay in the classroom and read rather than be teased on the playground for my various failures to fit in. I liked to sit and read and eat, and maybe my mother worried I'd grow sedentary and isolated. In an effort to give me more social structure, and with the hope that I'd both get exercise and build more confidence, my mother had signed me up for the swim team at the local Y when I was eleven years old, and I stuck with it all through middle school. I did love to swim, and I wasn't bad at it, but I had no talent for team sports. Gym class had been a series of humiliations for me: last kid picked for teams, "easy out" chanted when I walked to bat in a softball game. I'd drift as far off into the outfield as the teacher would allow.

At least with swimming I could remain pretty independent. You don't have to coordinate with other human bodies; you stay in your own lane. But our team practised constantly and I mostly hated these sessions. You're lazy, the coach told me. I often felt as if my arms and legs were made of heavy, stiff clay.

Swim meets were infused with the smell of chlorine in the same way that my mother's art school hallways were marked by the smell of turpentine. At meets, I would binge at the baked goods table on crispy cereal squares packed with M&M's and brownies made by other people's parents and sold cheap for quick energy. Instead of uniforms we wore warm-up sweats over our swimsuits. My mother bought me a thin navy-blue sweatpants-and-hoodie combo at JC Penney's and then embroidered the team's name on the sleeve. But she spelled it wrong: PIRANAHAS in yellow thread running down my arm.

"You know that's spelled wrong," people—kids, parents—would tell me.

"Yes, I know," I'd answer.

Years later, I read an old letter to my father in which my mother brags about me winning some race—but I don't remember that I even once came in second. Early on I became so disappointed at trying hard and coming in third or fourth that I started to intentionally throw my races, to slowly plod with an affected despondency as if I might sink to the bottom of the pool. My solution to the anxiety of competition was to give up in advance. But of course, this just made me feel like a bigger loser.

By eighth grade, boys had become a focus, a tool with which we tried to define our own value. Ours was a coed team, and we girls felt it was our job to oversee who had crushes on whom. Andrea and I decided we liked a shy, good-looking kid and tormented him for attention. We even named our pretend band after him by spelling his name backwards (not that we told him, or anyone, about the existence of our pretend band). On the day I met my father, my attention was fixed on this boy at a swim meet.

My father had driven to this neutral territory of the swim meet—it was not so far from where he lived, about a forty-five-minute drive away. My mother and father—to think of them as a unit, as "parents," felt wrong—sat across from each other at a long plastic table, the kind common to school lunchrooms, in a large room jammed full of families. By that time, my mother had not seen my father in more than eleven years.

My father had brought me a bag of things—presents, but not wrapped. In fact, they weren't presents at all, in the traditional sense. They appeared to be castoffs. A used jump rope that was way too long for me to use, alternating blue and yellow plastic tube segments along a rope, all scuffed. My father was into physical fitness, was there to support my sportiness. He had also included a used paperback of the novel *Vision Quest*. A while later I read it, because Madonna appears in a scene in the movie adaptation, and we were able to sneak-watch R-rated movies on cable at Andrea's house. The book was a strange choice to give an adolescent girl: it was a dark and sad story, and it had dark and sad sex in it. I remember the young man stuck between his sad, menopausal mother, grieving behind a closed door after a radical hysterectomy, and an older lover who had lost her child and whose breasts still leaked milk.

Later, Joanna admitted to me that although she had felt perfectly calm about meeting up with my father that day, the minute she saw him walk into the room and saw his face, "I wanted to pick something up and throw it at him."

But she didn't throw anything. The two of them were cordial, if stiff, in front of me. I came over and sat down with them, and shyly studied my father. I considered his dark beard, his pale skin, his blue eyes. This guy is my father. I repeated the word *father* in my head but couldn't grasp what it might mean for him and me.

The pressure inside me was too intense and I found I couldn't push myself through my race. I cut the water cleanly with my hands—I always had good form—but I wouldn't or couldn't try to go faster. It was a refusal to perform for him, as he watched beside my mother in the stands, but I took no pleasure in defiance, felt only shame in my loss. For years afterward I wondered if he would have made more of an effort to see me again if I had won. As it was, I didn't see him again for four years.

❦

WHILE I WAS writing this book, the guy my mother met in art school would email me random memories about Joanna. He told me that when I was a kid, he sometimes came over and rolled around on the floor, making out with my mother, after I fell asleep. He told me the story of Joanna breaking down in class when listening to the John Giorno poem. He told me a version of the sensed-presence story that she'd told me so many times. "She said she was washing the dishes and felt something flitting around her and brushing against her face like a butterfly. She felt it was some kind of spirit, and decided, 'I should give this thing a home.' That night you were conceived." It was strange reading this story in an email from someone I hadn't seen in more than forty years. I didn't know she had told anyone else this story. And I was irritated by the details he had wrong. She hadn't said anything to me about washing the dishes. But now I think: maybe it's me who has the details wrong. She had made me feel that the presence had been hanging around a long time before she'd extended an invitation to it. I had imagined she had even felt the presence before she arrived in California. I had imagined that I had saved her. This story is part of the reason I felt I belonged completely to my mother, and that whoever my father may have been didn't matter. It was always about her and me: how I found her, how she let me in.

Our team had two coaches: a nice assistant who would smile and say, "You're going to look just like your mom when you get older," and a mean coach, the one who called me lazy and yelled at my mother in front of everyone for being late with team fees, ordering me out of the pool once until she wrote a cheque to clear our balance. At our next practice after I met my father, the nice coach asked me, "Who was that guy with your mom at the meet on Saturday?" He stood above me in sweatpants on the wet deck of the pool as I held on to the edge of the deep-end, treading water.

"My father," I said.

"I've never seen him before," the coach remarked. He was fishing but trying to be casual, gentle.

"Me either," I said brightly, half smirking, half shrugging. *Haha.* And I pushed off from the wall with my feet, my palms pressed together and pointing toward the other side of the pool. I continued to laugh as I frog-kicked my body under the surface of the water for as long as possible before coming up again for air.

Hahahaha.

racket / radiance / radiation / raft / rage / raid
rail / rainwater / raise / rake / rampage
rancour / rank / rant / rape / rapidity / rapport
rapture / rash / rat / ration / rave / raven / reach
reaction / reader / reality / realm / realtor
reanimation / reason / rebel / receipts / reception
recipe / reciprocity / recitation / recklessness
reckoning / recognition / recollection
recommendation / reconstruction / recovery
recreation / redaction / redemption / reduction
reference / refinement / R E F L E C T I O N
refrain / refreshment / refrigerator / refuge
refusal / regeneration / regret / regulation
rehabilitation / reincarnation / reinforcements
rejection / relapse / relationship / relatives
religion / remark / remembrance / reminder
repetition / repression / repulsion / requests
resentments / reservoir / residue / resilience
resolve / resources / rest / restoration / restriction
results / reverberation / reversal / revolution
rhapsody / rhizome / rhubarb / rhyme / rhythm
ribbons / richness / riddle / rigamarole / rigour
ring / ripple / risk / rite / rival / river / road
role / rollercoaster / romance / roof / room
roots / rope / roses / rot / roulette / route
routine / row / rubbish / rubble / ruin
rules / rupture / rush / rust

FOR YEARS WHEN I was a child, people told me that I was going to grow into the spitting image of my mother. By the time I turned fourteen, people told me that I already had.

Joanna and I could fit into the same clothes, although she didn't approve of me borrowing her things. When she wasn't looking, I'd sneak into her bedroom and spray myself with her French perfume. I carried around her Signet paperback edition of Whitman's *Leaves of Grass*, the one with a soft illustration of the bearded bard in muted colours, because she'd told me she had carried it around when she was fourteen. I dragged my first boyfriend to the art museum and insisted we kiss below the wrought iron spiral staircase, the exact spot where she had once kissed her first boyfriend. My kiss—which was with the lead from our high school production of *Bye Bye Birdie*, a dorky junior to my dorky freshman—was disappointing, staged and mechanical. But there was something in my idea of my mother that I was hungry to inhabit, even if I couldn't quite catch up to it.

When I started high school, Joanna wrote to my father, thanking him for money he had sent—a cheque every Christmas—and updating him on how I was doing in school. She wrote, "I was not made to be the mother of a teenager." But she also wrote, "She got an A in Geometry. A lot can be forgiven for an A in Geometry."

After eighth grade, so that I could go to a better-rated high school, my mother and I moved back closer to my grandparents. At first we had a cramped apartment behind Sunshine Foods. The following year my grandmother helped my mother buy a house, around the block from my grandparents. Our house was situated next door to the house directly behind my grandparents' house, so the corners of our square-lot backyards touched. My grandfather built what my grandmother called a stile—my grandmother loved using the word *stile*—sturdy wooden steps that made it possible to climb out of one yard and into the other, right over the fence. We popped back and forth, carrying leftovers and loaves of bread.

Joanna continued dating, although, as in our previous homes, she rarely had a serious boyfriend for very long. When I was thirteen years old and my mother was thirty-five, she had a boyfriend, Richard, who was twenty-five. I did the math and realized he was right between our ages. They had met at the Y, where he was on the adult swim team. He wasn't bad-looking, but he wasn't great-looking, and I remember he was already losing his hair. They dated for close to a year.

I liked Richard at first, but after a while he began to make little comments about my appearance, and remarked how one of his friends had been hoping I was older than I was—"legal," he said, laughing. At that, my mother's lips pressed together so hard they went white. The summer after I graduated eighth grade, before we had moved, Joanna, Richard and I all watched the Fourth of July fireworks on a blanket on the grassy curb across from the golf course. Richard began rubbing my back, and soon my muscles became so tense that my body ached painfully wherever he touched me.

One day after school I was alone in the house—Joanna arrived home at five o'clock every day—and the phone rang. It was Richard. We talked for a long time. It felt a little strange, but I'd never had anyone take such an interest in me. I was still on the phone with him, in my mother's bedroom, on the bed where she was reading George Bernard Shaw's *Pygmalion* to me every night, when she arrived home from work. Joanna heard the tone of my voice—giggly, hushed—and realized it was Richard on the other end. She flew into a rage. She was furious with him. And although she never talked to me directly about it, I knew she was furious with me. Not long after that, they broke up. It was around the same time I got my first period, an event that also seemed to anger her.

Even many years later, if Richard's name came up, my mother would scowl. *Oh him. What an asshole.*

❦

THERE WASN'T ANYONE steady after that for a couple of years, until my mother started dating a guy she met at her twentieth high school reunion. The two of them hadn't been friends in high school, but now, in 1987, they were both single and they hit it off. He was vaguely entrepreneurial, the sort of guy who paid for things in cash—he even paid for his cars in cash. He drove a Corvette and lived in a new-money suburb about twenty minutes away from us, but at the same time he didn't seem rich, exactly. My mom and I didn't know how he made his money. I still don't, to this day. It bothered my mother that she didn't know, but it didn't bother her enough to stop seeing him.

This guy was crafty and liked to tinker with things, although there was usually something not quite right about everything he made. He made my mother a clock out of a bevelled diamond-shaped mirror that slowly stopped working. He built me an aquarium that poisoned seven fish in a row. I'd find them floating on the surface of the water, eating each other, their flesh rotting. I got along with him well enough, but he often grated on my nerves. To be fair, by this point I was fifteen, and everything grated on my nerves.

"So was my mom cool in high school?" I asked him once, smirking. "She's always talking about how she went to go see the MC5 play the Grande Ballroom, how she hung out downtown. She says she was cool."

He looked at my mother and raised his eyebrows.

"I never said that!" she protested. "I never said I was cool!"

Certainly, I wasn't cool. I didn't know how to dress, and I borderline worshipped all of the older girls who seemed to believe in themselves. I looked up to the punks, who dyed their hair and wore layers of ripped and shredded textiles, a hint of soot glinting in their shadowy glamour as they clustered by the lockers closest to the doors so that they could get out of school fast. I looked up to the cheerleaders, rich girls who smoked pot and wore coloured contacts and always looked clean. Impossibly clean. I admired some of the burnouts, who also smoked pot, but were not rich; they wore thick black eyeliner and took no shit. All of these kids, regardless of where they fit, seemed fearless to me.

I tried wearing hand-me-downs from friends, but I assembled the pieces in bizarre combinations: torn jeans with moccasins and a peacoat. I wanted to be a part of everything. Once, I got wasted on two cans of Budweiser (like my mother, I had no tolerance for alcohol) and danced with the Hare Krishnas at Hart Plaza, my hair in braids, around my neck a blue string with an *om* sign carved in sandalwood that I found in my mother's jewellery box. I spun and spun in the Krishnas' circle, clapping and chanting and laughing. I dismissed with a friendly shrug the earnest missionary who approached me. Later, a guy I met through my friends tentatively flirted with me. "Weren't you dancing with the Hare Krishnas?" he asked, clearly suspicious. I laughed and laughed as the night's bright spark burned toward black.

In my senior year, I painted my room an unfortunate purple, put my mattress on the floor and covered it with my mother's old memory quilt. I listened to Joni Mitchell's *Blue*. Joanna would often spend the night at her boyfriend's place, and I would invite my friends over, and we would drink wine coolers and call guys we liked.

❦

MANY DAYS, AFTER school, a fog would come over me. I would lie on my bed and stare at the wall and think. And think. And think. Sometimes exciting ideas formed in my head. Other times, though, I just thought about the guys who liked to get together and listen to Frank Zappa and watch *It's Garry Shandling's Show.*

Joanna didn't approve of my behaviour. She'd read my diary and learned that what she feared was true: I was drinking, and I was messing around with boys. She grounded me for two months. Meanwhile, the fog continued. It would come over me in a rush, and I'd feel my body become numb. I became faceless, and I would binge-eat or binge-drink to quiet the grinding anxiety, gratefully sinking into darkness.

My experiments with alcohol helped block the fog for stretches of time. It seemed to dull my neural receptors and drop me into an abyss I experienced as pure relief. Sometimes, my friend Andrea and I would manage to buy cheap champagne, a brand called André that we bought in honour of a guy she obsessed over. He had long hair and worked at Noir Leather, a store that sold all things studded. André went to Andrea's high school, and we had swooned when we heard him sing a song by the band Ratt at a talent show. Later, he would achieve low-level celebrity by landing a spot on the first season of *The Real World.* So we'd drink pink André champagne and eat chocolate-covered raisins that my mother bought us, while listening to REM and Peter Gabriel records and talking about boys. Joanna had painted our living room the colour of Pepto-Bismol, and our drinks matched the walls.

One of my boyfriends in high school felt my mother competed with me. In hindsight, I think he found Joanna a little creepy, though I couldn't have expressed it that way at the time. For all that my mother frustrated me, and for all that I strained against her, I still romanticized her. At seventeen, I never questioned her appeal. Although some of my male friends had crushes on her and she flirted with my boyfriends—she flirted with everyone—this never bothered me. It was just how she talked to men; it was like wallpaper I'd never noticed. But it did bother some of my boyfriends. I understand now that she probably needed to know that young men saw her as beautiful, desirable. And they did. My friend Art—I ended up going to prom with him when his date dumped him at the last minute—thought she looked like Jessica Lange.

❦

DURING THIS TIME, I had a number of jobs. For one month I waitressed at a restaurant called Sign of the Beefcarver. The uniform was a white nurse's dress and shoes worn with a red gingham bonnet and matching half apron. We servers would carry cafeteria-style trays of sliced beast or liver and onions to tables of seniors, who tipped in quarters. After that, my cousin Ann hooked me up with a job at a tanning salon and weight-loss centre called Bodyshapers, where I wrapped people head to toe in mud-soaked bandages. I also worked at a fancy shoe boutique run by a German woman with a Louise Brooks haircut. I vividly remember her pointing out to a customer that my black grosgrain pumps with a Louis XIV heel—the one indulgence I had allowed myself out of the money I was saving for university—would have been much cuter paired with coloured tights instead of the tan pantyhose I had on. The customer to whom she'd said this made a face at me that said *sorry*. But my boss was right, of course. I still was figuring out how to dress myself, what kind of girl to be.

The best job I had was working for a woman who ran her own small vintage clothing store. It wasn't the coolest store in town, but it was definitely the coolest place I had ever worked.

My boss liked to push the edges of her relationships with people. She made me cry once, when she told me that my allegiance to my mother meant I wasn't taking my father's side of the story into consideration. I shook with anger. "He left! She raised me!"

"You don't know what happened," she said coolly as she lit a cigarette. "You only know your mother's version."

I cried about this later to my boyfriend, but he couldn't understand why I cared what a woman in her thirties, who wore big earrings and too much makeup, thought about anything. "She's just like somebody's aunt," he said.

My boss loved being behind the counter, perched on her stool in her store, chain-smoking menthols. There, she was imperious. Both the counter and the stool were high, so that she'd peer down at me as she asked me to fetch her things from various corners of the small store.

One day, Joanna came to visit me at the store and my boss told us a story about how she had been violently attacked and raped by a stranger when she was younger.

After we left together, my mother brooded a bit. She couldn't understand how my boss had so casually told her story to someone she barely knew. Joanna was suspicious. Then she said: "I was raped, and I've never told anyone about it."

"What are you talking about? When?"

"I don't want to talk about it," my mother said. The lid of a heavy box snapping shut. "I'm serious, Damian. I'm not going to talk about it."

"Mom! You can't just drop something like that," I said. "How old were you?"

"Fifteen. And I'm not going to talk about it."

We kept walking to the car. We walked down the street in Royal Oak. We walked down the street in East Lansing, we walked down the street in Ann Arbor, we walked down the street in London, in Paris. We walked down the street in Chicago. I kept moving, and so did she. And everywhere we went, men smiled at us and said, *Like sisters, you two must be sisters.*

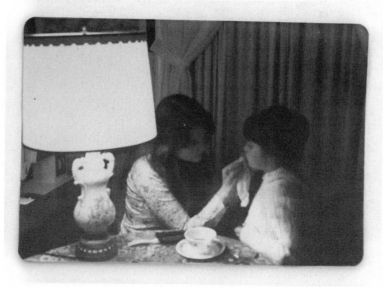

HALLOWEEN 1977
Joanna and me, in my grandparents' dining room

oak / oasis / oath / obedience / obelisk
obfuscation / obituary / objectification / objection
objectives / obligation / obliteration / oblivion
obliviousness / obscenity / obscurity / obstacle
occasion / occlusion / occult / occupation
occurrence / O C E A N / oddness / odour
offense / official / oil / omen / omission
onslaught / ontogeny / opacity / opal / opening
operative / opponent / opposites / oppression
optimism / ordeal / orders / organ / organization
orientation / origin / orphan / ostracization
outlet / outrage / outside / overdraft / overseer
overture / owl / oxytocin

kitchen table

t.v.

frying pan

chairs

mop and
bucket

dishwashing
liquid

ramen
noodles,
canned soups,
bread

loyalty

refrigerator
magnets

jams, tea

coffee

Bed

dresser

desk

lamps

scrubby
sponge

rocking chair

bath thingys

spices

cooking stuff

shoe polish

silver polish

I want the
winter to be
over

MY NOTEBOOK,
CHICAGO, 1995

IN 1995, I made a list of everything I needed for my first apartment in Chicago.

After graduating from university and living in London, England, for a year, I had travelled solo through Europe on a train pass before heading back to the States, smoking cheap cigarettes and drawing imaginary floor plans for my future Chicago apartment. I had toured Peggy Guggenheim's house on the Grand Canal in Venice and had stood before *Setting for a Fairy Tale* by Joseph Cornell: a thick forest of white-painted branches looming behind the image of a palace. In this piece, I recognized something I couldn't articulate, something that suggested my home would always be a dream. I arrived back at the Detroit airport sporting an embarrassing mid-Atlantic accent I couldn't even hear in my own voice; the customs officer grilled me about where I was born, and when I finally advanced through the line, my mother laughed at my indignation. "You sound British!" she said. I knew by then that I'd only be in Michigan for a short time, just long enough to save some money. An ex-boyfriend of my mother's offered me a job at the counter of the used-car dealership he managed. Two months later I was on my way to Chicago. It had never occurred to me to stay in Detroit.

Earlier that year, my mother had visited me in London, and we'd spent a weekend with another friend of mine in Paris. The pattern had been set: I would move to a new city and my mother would see it for the first time through me.

Surprisingly, it was my father who helped me move the last of my belongings to Chicago. I'd started seeing him every few months while I was at university. He told me his wife was more comfortable now with him seeing me, since I no longer lived with my mother. I had been torn: I was angry with him, but I also wanted to know him. He told me once that he'd never had a relationship as intense as the one he'd had with my mother. When I reported this back to her, her eyes narrowed. "That's because no one has ever made me as angry as your father did," she said. Nonetheless, she had remained reasonably friendly with him in the years that followed their breakup.

Now my father arrived at her house and we loaded up his minivan. This was one of the few times I ever saw them in the same room together. They were polite to each other, but later she said to me, "Just so you know, he was a lot better-looking when I was with him."

My furniture in Chicago consisted of a mustard-yellow velour couch that had been in my grandparents' basement, a futon I bought, and the Formica kitchen table and chairs left behind by the former tenant, a woman who worked with my friend Brett at Reckless Records. My father slept on the couch in my new living room that night, then drove back the next day to the small town in Michigan where he lived. It was the last time I would see him for nearly twenty years.

Finally, my life was beginning. In my notebook, I made plans of self-improvement and goals for who I might be.

Not long after I moved to Chicago, the much younger guy my mother had been dating back in Michigan dumped her. I'd never seen her so hurt, and I fantasized about going back to Michigan, finding the dumb smoke-free bar he liked and throwing a drink in his face. "That's for my mother," I'd say, as if I was an actor in an eighties nighttime soap.

My mother almost never drank, but she had kept a bottle of vodka in her freezer because this boyfriend liked it. After he broke her heart, she pulled out the bottle one night and drank by herself. And then she called me. I was still living alone, and I felt patient with her. I liked being the strong one. I liked being the one to comfort her. She kept saying, "And I thought, I'll call my baby," over and over. The next day she rang with a brutal hangover. She had impulsively decided to drive to Chicago to see me. She needed me. She was leaving right now, she said.

The minute I got off the phone with my mother, I began deep cleaning my apartment. When Joanna arrived five hours later, she couldn't believe how clean it was. But I wanted her to see me flourishing. I knew she might worry about the neighbourhood and my hand-to-mouth lifestyle—my first year in Chicago I made $11,000—and I wanted to make sure she wouldn't try to convince me to do things differently. In any case, I wouldn't have listened to her, and I think she knew that. We simply enjoyed each other's company for a few days.

MY MOTHER NEVER had another serious boyfriend after that, though she continued to date casually.

"It's the nature of the species to pair up," she told me when I visited her soon after, as we sat together on her bed. Her French perfume bottle, a gift from a married lover she hadn't seen in years, was still on her antique vanity. She also told me, after burning a copy of the novel *The Bridges of Madison County* on the hibachi grill in the garage, that she had decided to move to Florida, where her father, my grandfather, had just moved. (My grandmother had died from her cancer three years before, and my grandfather had found it impossible to stay in their house without her.) Joanna's brother Roger also lived there with his wife and their extended family.

I thought my mother was reacting to her breakup and advised her to wait six months to see if she still wanted to make the move. She told me she'd considered moving to Chicago, but she wasn't confident I was going to stick around. I saw this as a bullet dodged. I didn't want her to move to Chicago. And although it was nice having her live five hours away, I wasn't upset at the idea of her moving to Florida. I just thought she should make sure she really wanted to go, that she wasn't uprooting herself on a whim. She listened to me, and waited. Six months later she told me, "I still want to go."

ONCE JOANNA LANDED in Florida, her new life fell into place quickly. She found a job designing ads for a trade magazine serving the produce business and began to make more money than she ever had. And she had done well selling the house in the Detroit suburbs. She still lived frugally, mostly out of habit, but now she had enough extra income to be very generous with me. She paid for my plane tickets to visit her, took me out to dinner and splurged on a couple of vacations for us. On one trip we drifted around Key West, checked out the six-toed cats at Hemingway's house, ate conch fritters at Jimmy Buffett's Margaritaville and drank big, brightly coloured cocktails every couple of hours, never getting drunk. For her fiftieth birthday, we spent the weekend at Disney World.

❧

THESE ARE MY favourite memories of my mother and me in Florida: We're in bikinis, soaking in the condo hot tub together at night. Above us is a crescent moon, while below the surface of the bubbling water are lights that make the green-painted walls glow. I think of European frescoes. Back in her living room, I demand that my mother bring me a beer. She asks me to repeat myself, confused. "You heard me," I say. "Bring me a beer." She disappears into the bathroom. When she comes back, she hands me a small mirror.

Soon after she moved to Florida, my mother found a beach of her own. I can imagine myself there, beside her again, so easily. The beach was part of a park, a nature preserve full of banyan trees and overgrowth and uneven ground. The beach itself was small and more dirt than sand, with the exposed roots of the trees extending nearly to the waterline. It was a wild and raw bit of shore, and we were the only people on it.

This was nothing like the Fort Lauderdale beach, with its miles-long row of parked cars stretched along the coast, young tanned bodies parked on parallel towels as far as the eye could see. I hated all of that. I detested the sunglasses people wore there—black plastic fronts with neon-coloured arms. I hated the hardened comb tracks through the gel in the guys' hair, the gold chains, the sunny, shiny, high gloss of it all. I rejected the whole package—not just the superficiality of the surfaces, but the submission to that relentless light, the embrace of a bald, humiliating exposure to a numbing, unbroken blast of sunshine. I wanted shadow. I wanted to disappear into a city night, not into a mass of squirming, voiceless flesh that promised only obliteration, the annihilation of nuance.

After walking through the landscape on my mother's beach, she and I sit on our towels in the silty sand and watch the waves roll in. The hypnotic rhythm of those waves slowly erodes my internal chatter about myself. From the coolness beneath the trees, I study how the water lifts up in a swell, building until it reaches its peak, how the green underbelly of the wave is covered over by the white, foaming crest diving back into itself. It's like watching a large, beautiful, dangerous animal breathe, doing its work of staying alive. The pattern washes my brain out, my anxieties and fears and frustrations and worries replaced with a looping, low-toned drone. My mother and I fall into a comfortable silence, side by side, staring forward into eternity.

"I love it here," she says.

IT WAS IN Chicago that I met my future husband, Mike, and fell in love. Mike was tall and good-looking and had beautiful eyes. He was quick and funny and kind—so kind. He was also disciplined and made sacrifices to do the thing he loved to do—make music. He worked his ass off, but always wanted to do better. He took care of himself, and soon he took care of me. He believed I could do anything. In fact, he was all in from the moment we met. Back then I was messy, but I picked a steady guy. And I grabbed on to him, and never let go.

After we had been dating a year, Mike visited me while I was staying with my mother in Florida over Christmas vacation. It was unsettling seeing her through his eyes. His parents, married since the early 1960s, were independent, accomplished citizens of the world. My mother spoke in baby talk. Like her flirting, this was something I didn't even notice until someone else drew my attention to it. One morning, announcing she was about to take a "show-show" (her cutesy abbreviation of the word shower), she asked if either of us needed to "go potty." After she left the room, Mike looked at me and mouthed, "Potty?!" I rolled my eyes and shrugged.

One night when we were alone, Mike said to me, "I'm not trying to be mean, but your father must have been really smart. Because, you're really smart and your mother—"

"She's a lot smarter than she acts," I told him. I never thought Joanna was dumb, though everyone treated her as if she was.

I think my mother picked up on Mike's impressions. It was important to her that he know she was clever and resourceful.

Joanna started flexing. She talked about how often she practised piano, how she listened to French-language radio when she worked. Mike and my mother bonded over a shared enthusiasm for crossword puzzles.

"I do crosswords every day. I'll never get Alzheimer's," she told him, beaming.

table / tableau / taboo / tack / tackle / tactic / tail
talc / tale / talisman / talk / tally / tambourine
tangle / tank / tantrum / tape / target / task / taste
tax / tea / tears / teat / technique / technology
teen / telepathy / telephone / television / tell
tempest / tempo / temptation / tenant / tenderness
tension / tentacle / termination / terrain / terror
test / testament / testimony / texture / theatre
theme / therapy / thief / thimble / thistle / thorn
thread / threat / threnody / threshold / throat
thumb / thunder / thyroid / tide / timbre / time
tinsel / tit / title / toad / tobacco / toddler
togetherness / toil / toilet / tolerance / toll
tomato / tone / tongue / tool / torch / torment
tornado / torture / touch / T O W E R / toxin
toy / traces / trade / train / trance / transaction
transference / transformation / transgression
transience / transit / transition / translation
transmission / transparency / transplant
transportation / trap / trash / trauma / travel
travesty / tray / tread / treason / treasure / treat
treatment / trees / tremor / trend / trespass
triage / trials / triangulation / tribute / trick
trifle / trigger / trilogy / trimester / trip / tripe
triumph / trouble / truce / trunk / trust / truth
tryst / tumour / tune / turbulence / turf
turmoil / turncoat / turpentine / turquoise / tush
tussle / tweezers / twilight / twin / twinge
twinkle / twist / twosome / typo

4 WAYS TO GET HIS
ATTENTION—NOW!

5 SIGNS HE REALLY
LIKES YOU

6 SNEAKY WAYS TO MEET
ROCK STARS

183 WAYS TO BE A
PARTY GODDESS

301 WAYS TO LOOK HOT
FOR THE HOLIDAYS

547 WAYS TO LOOK
AMAZING THIS FALL

THE 4 QUESTIONS YOU
CAN'T ASK ANYONE:
ANSWERED

THOUGH I WAS living in the East Village; though I woke up that morning and walked to the R line near Cooper Union, which was beside the Kmart where I'd recently bought a bunch of deadstock Fruit of the Loom men's underwear that I'd tie-dyed blue for no reason; though I exited the subway at Columbus Circle and walked past however many people to arrive at the Hearst Building; though I entered the crowded elevator and rode it to the lobby of the teen fashion magazine where I worked, a lobby decorated with leopard-print carpet, zebra-striped walls and a hot-pink lipstick-scrawled logo; though I walked through the office and past most of my co-workers to reach my private, small, windowless workspace in the copy department, it was my mother—not my colleagues, not the people in the elevator or on the street or on the subway—who delivered the news to me that two planes had flown into the World Trade Center.

"Oh my god, thank god you're okay," she said breathlessly through the receiver when I answered the phone on my desk. I'd barely set down my purse, had yet to go pour myself a cup of coffee.

"What are you talking about? What's wrong?" I asked.

"Damian!" she said sharply.

I walked out of my dark office into the larger maze of grey cubicles. A junior editor nearby was glued to a transistor radio. She told me a plane had just crashed into the Pentagon.

A fact-checker approached me a little later, lowering her voice. "I realize this is a shitty thing to say, but god, you know this is all we're going to hear about for months."

♥

MIKE AND I had been in New York for more than a year, after he'd lived with me in Chicago for nine months. We'd moved to New York because he had a rent-controlled apartment in a cool neighbourhood, because he had convinced me that "everyone should live in New York for a couple of years," and because I had come to the end of the line in Chicago. I wanted to start over. Again. I loved starting over. So I gave up my prestigious, if low-paying, editorial position where I was paid to read poetry. My problem with working at a literary journal was that I read submissions all day, and then was unable to write a word myself in the evenings. In Chicago I had a cool job and interesting artist friends, yet I found I couldn't make anything of my own.

I had a theory that if I found a decent-paying job I didn't

"take home with me," I'd free up my creative energy. I jumped at the chance to work at a teen fashion magazine. My mother and I had always loved to read glossy, chatty magazines. It was a guilty pleasure for me by my late twenties, but a pleasure nonetheless. It will be hilarious, I thought. It will be a scream, I thought. And then I'll go home and write poems, I thought.

Free Hanson stickers. Free Britney stickers. Make your ex-boyfriend want you back. Look hot tonight. Clothes! Hair! Makeup! Kissing tricks to drive him crazy. Real girls. Your crush. Are you annoying? Get that guy.

I loved my dark cave of an office—although it was barely a couple of feet larger than my desk—because it had a door. Outside that door was the copy department, which consisted of two rows of cubicles that filled up with freelance copy editors for two weeks of every month, when we were "shipping." Shipping was what we called hell: twelve- to sixteen-hour days during which you might read the same cover story about Justin Timberlake or Jessica Simpson ten times. All of the individual pieces that made up each issue—fashion spreads, celebrity features, Boy-o-meter, Ouch!, Hey!, His Diary, etc.—circulated separately in their own large blue folders. Once the production department set the page in layout, a piece moved through many hands before it was sent to the printer: the designer, the assigned editor, a fact-checker, a copy editor, the deputy editor, the executive editor, the editor in chief. Each person was assigned a colour-coded writing instrument so that it was easy to know whose comments were whose, from the tight red pencil of fact-checking to the expressive hot-pink cursive of our EIC. "Not funny enough!" would appear next to a lacklustre photo caption. The price of a pair of heart-covered panties had changed, the apostrophe in the band name 'NSync was pointing the wrong way, or the hyphen in Blink-182 was missing. My job was to make sure that all the corrections were made, that the page was clean and perfect and ready for our reader, a girl like I had been, in suburban Wherever, who would laugh at the embarrassing stories about someone caught buying tampons in front of her crush. Periods were always *super-embarrassing*. (Our style guide had a list of when to compound words following the prefix *super* and when to hyphenate.)

On my desk sat a pile of blue folders and printouts of the "map," which showed where each story was placed in the issue. Every time the stories shuffled around, we all received a new map. One of my tasks was to draw a big X through the squares that represented each story that had been finalized. I had a giant computer monitor on my desk, too, so that I could see what I was doing as I entered changes. I spent a lot of my time tracking the "kerning," the space between characters, to make a line fit and keep the "rag" pretty. The rag is the shape that the unjustified right side of a text column makes on the page. The art director, a beautiful, ambitious artist from California whose office I liked to hide out in, hated an ugly rag.

Everyone in that office was beautiful—even the people who were treated like wallflowers were objectively attractive—and nearly everyone was under the age of thirty. I'd never worked in a more homogeneous environment in my life. Though the editor in chief was Iranian-American and the magazine included far more models and subjects of colour than had ever appeared in the pages of teen mags when I was growing up, the industry remained overwhelmingly white. A Black friend of mine, working then as a part-time fact-checker, shrugged at her decision to walk away from her previous job as an assistant beauty editor at a popular makeup mag. "Nobody looked like me," she said. Almost all of the beauty editors at the turn of the millennium were white, blue-eyed blondes. If they hadn't been born blond, then they saw someone about that, and if their hair had a wave, they saw someone to iron that wave out. I found the pressure to conform insidious; it crept in like a virus. Most of the women, especially those at the top of the masthead, wore three-inch heels every day. The uniform was a fancy top, maybe a fake-vintage Duran Duran T-shirt, worn with a pair of 7 jeans that flared slightly over a pair of pointy-toed heels. At editorial meetings we pulled compliments for each other out of a Grin Box, a practice borrowed from someone's sorority. When the economy started to falter and budgets constricted, a suit from HQ came to speak to us. They had discovered the company had been spending thousands of dollars annually so that editors could send each other congratulatory floral bouquets: we were ordered to stop sending ourselves flowers. Also newly forbidden was the popular practice of burning giant perfumed candles at our desks. Apparently someone had realized that stacks of loose paper, distracted editors and open flames were a bad mix.

What I loved most about my job was the smug pleasure that fixing a sentence gave me. It made me feel smart that I knew where to place the comma in a caption. I became addicted to that sense of superiority, the idea that I was "better at words" than the writers, though what I longed to do was actually write. I resented my co-workers who wrote features on fun things to do during spring break, even if I did catch them crying over these same articles in the bathroom. It was like we were all transported back to high school. A part of me still wanted to be the cheerleader, *and* the Ivy League–bound preppie, *and* the punk with my locker closest to the doors. But I had never been any of these girls; I had always drifted between them, adjusting my face based on who was looking at it. I stayed in the job, gnashing my teeth, judging everyone, hating myself.

I remember an article on toxic friendships, and one of the frenemy archetypes to avoid was described as the "Negativa." The Negativa was cutting, self-protected, untrustworthy. The Negativa was a bitch. The Negativa's only point-of-view was side-eye. I remember thinking, The Negativa is me.

Living in New York was a challenge. I missed my Chicago friends. Mike was constantly on the road, playing drums in two bands and flying from the end of one tour to the beginning of another one. I was lonely all the time and furious at him for doing what he loved and paradoxically fixated on the idea of getting married. All the women I worked with were serious about their diamond and platinum engagement rings. Those rings, I began to think, sparkled in an undeniably pretty way. I started to want a pair of 7 jeans.

Despite my glowering angst, I genuinely liked my colleagues. And I admired the editor in chief; we were the same age, but I couldn't imagine shouldering her responsibilities. The amount of pressure on her to perform everything perfectly was inconceivable to me, and she worked harder than anyone I'd ever seen. But I knew I was also sliding into a sullen-teenager pose. I might as well have been smoking menthols against the brick wall behind the school, picking at my chipped black nail polish. Looking back, I see how easy it was to be smug, how cheap. Even now, taking shots at the culture of a teen fashion magazine feels less like an attack on the machinery of female conditioning and more like just another form of misogyny. I'd heard editors from general interest magazines refer to this end of the industry as "the pink ghetto." But I also remember a colleague pointing out to me that these magazines were still the only publications that regularly reported on new medical studies relating to women's health. Our magazine tackled issues such as rape, substance abuse and cutting, and this was long before Google became a verb, a time when teen magazines were the main source of information for girls scared about STDs or getting pregnant, who were feeling depressed or excluded.

The thrill I derived from fixing a sentence, correcting inconsistencies of style, was related to my magnetic attraction to the cyclical promises magazine cover lines offered readers every month. Every month, a fresh blueprint to transformation, a roadmap to confidence, to the ever-elusive *fix*. My mother and I were both devotees to the grinding, unstoppable engine of self-improvement. The right life was always just around the corner, a couple of tips away.

Joanna was proud of my job in New York, and she bragged about it. She loved that my job impressed her bosses in Florida at the produce magazine. "They say you're in the Big Time," she told me.

It wasn't a good fit for me, but instead of quitting and finding a job that suited me better, I slunk around muttering, dragging my rain cloud behind me. One of my more disgruntled colleagues, sharing my inner turmoil, turned me on to kundalini yoga and introduced me to her guru/masseur, a muscular fifty-year-old former coke dealer. In our first session, he put his hands on my back and asked, "Why are you so mad at your mother?"

"What? No, I'm mad at my father," I told him.

He didn't agree. Later, I read a profile of him in another glossy mag. A famous actress who was also a client breathlessly explained how he had cut straight to the heart of her issues in their first session. "He asked me why I was so mad at my mother," she told the interviewer, "and immediately I knew he was right."

My office at work filled up with an eclectic collection of graff I'd scored off the table where editors threw freebies they didn't want to keep. A metal spider-like head massager. A cheerful Hello Kitty clock that ticked louder than any movie bomb as it marked off each passing second. A pair of Bulgari sunglasses. So much makeup and vanilla-scented body shimmer, and perfumes that were designed to smell like Snow, or Clean Laundry. One day the deputy editor showed me a small jar of soil she had been sent, with elegant lettering that read DIRT on the label. "This is so New York," she said.

❦

THE NIGHT OF September 10, 2001, Mike had left on a night flight to England to start a UK tour, so I was alone on the morning of the 11th. Years later, after my mother had become sick, she'd often tell Mike and me a story of how she'd rushed to my side the minute the news of the Twin Towers broke.

"I told the people 'I have to go see my baby' and they let me go!" she would say.

We didn't bother correcting her. The truth was, weeks passed before she was able to fly to New York from Boca.

IT FELT TO me as if I'd moved to New York at the wrong time in history—all of my romantic associations of the city were rooted in black-and-white photos of the Warhol Factory scene, or the early punk scene at CBGBs and Max's Kansas City, or even the colourful quirk of downtown life as depicted by *Desperately Seeking Susan*. But instead of living out my art-life fantasy, I felt like an extra on the set of *Sex and the City*. Everything seemed shiny and shallow.

At a friend's birthday party the summer after the towers came down, I found myself sunk deep into a couch, squished between an artist famous for one single photograph that incited the ire of the censorious senator Jesse Helms and a small, intense European who may as well have been wearing a monocle. The photographer was trying to cajole me into leaving the party for an after-hours club. The room was blue-lit and smoky, and I felt as if I were watching my companions through a layer of thick aquarium glass. I probably looked passive—exuding the perfect amount of out-of-it to attract a pickup attempt—but I knew I wasn't going anywhere with these creeps. The European was poking at my dress, feeling the synthetic floral fabric between his fingers, an appraiser. "Who makes this dress, where did you get it? Is it Marni?" he demanded.

"I ordered it from a website that advertises in teen fashion magazines," I told him, nursing my drink. My eyelids felt heavy.

"No!" he said, recoiling in disgust. "Why did you tell me that? You've ruined it."

He asked me how long I'd lived in New York, and then he told me a story: the anecdote about the frog.

"If you drop a live frog in a pot of boiling water, he will leap right out of the pot," he told me. "But if you place a frog in a pan of lukewarm water and slowly and steadily raise the temperature until the water begins to boil, the frog will stay in that pot until he is completely cooked."

The two men pressed against me on either side, while a glass coffee table in front of us made escape difficult. I imagined that if someone were to take a photo of us, the little vampire on my left wouldn't even show up on the film.

"That is what it is to live in New York City," the European finished with a flourish as he poked me in the arm again, hard enough to leave a small, dark bruise.

It's time to leave this party, I thought. It's time to get out of here.

saboteur / sacredness / sacrifice / sadness / safety
salary / sale / salt / salvation / sand / sandalwood
sandpaper / sandpiper / sapphire / sarcasm / satin
satire / satisfaction / saturation / scale / scan
scandal / scarab / scarlet / scenery / school
scorpion / scoundrel / scowl / scratch / scream
sculpture / seal / seashells / seclusion
S E C R E T S / security / sedative / seduction
seed / seesaw / senility / sense / sensitivity
sensuality / separation / sequence / seraph
serotonin / service / settlement / sex / shadow
shape / shard / shark / sheen / sheets / shellac
sherry / shield / shift / shimmer / shipwreck
shock / shoe / shore / sibling / sickness / sign
signifier / silence / silhouette / silk / silver / simile
sincerity / siren / sisters / skate / skills / skull / slip
smell / smile / smoke / snake / snapdragon / snow
solace / solution / song / soot / sorcery / sorrow
sound / sources / space / spark / spectre / speech
speed / spell / spider / stability / star / static
stencil / stitch / storm / story / strawberry / street
stress / stroke / structure / stuff / style
sublimation / submission / subterfuge
subterranean / suffering / suffocation / suggestion
sunshine / support / surname / surprise
surrender / surrogate / survivor / suspension
sweat / swimmer / swing / symmetry / sympathy
symptoms / synchronicity / system

MOVING TO CANADA did not immediately solve all of my problems. I had been depressed before the events of September 11; after them, a bone-deep fear, which had been following me all my life and was further enflamed by radio announcements about "orange alerts," now reached paranoiac levels. When my anxiety became too intense, I would binge-drink, drowning my thoughts for at least a few hours. I never started out to get drunk, but I ended up on the dark side of that knife's edge more than I wanted to admit. It felt good, the edges of my body blurring and dissolving.

Mike and I had moved, somewhat impulsively, to an apartment in Toronto recently vacated by friends. Another new start. The problem was, I brought my fear with me. I had no clear plans for my next career move, so I ended up working part-time at a health food store. I hung out with our neighbour upstairs and talked about ideas for creative projects I never started, like a horror movie shot in the country, or a piece of cinéma-vérité nonsense based on my wild female friends. I thought it would be funny to build a short story out of the names of guys and the track lists of the mixed tapes they'd made to woo and/or improve me—BRIAN: The Stranglers, Camper Van Beethoven, Pere Ubu; THOMAS: Scott Walker, Nick Drake, Syd Barrett; GORDON: Polvo, Bedhead, Guided by Voices; CLARK: The Cure, The Birthday Party, proto-emo something-something. But I didn't write stories or poems, I didn't make movies. I bit my nails and spun my wheels and threw bacchanalian dinner parties for the other "band wives" when Mike was on the road. American Thanksgiving, Lunar New Year—my wild female friends came over and we smoked and drank and lit sparklers and ran around the backyard whooping, wearing 1950s cocktail dresses, ripped slips and second-hand heels. We dressed up for each other, and we blurred out together, clutching each other and lurching into the void.

My mother developed the habit of timing her visits to coincide with Mike's trips out of town. This way, she didn't intrude on my time with Mike, which in those years of heavy touring was often brief—a few days here, a week or two there. She also got me all to herself; she liked Mike, but she preferred to see me one on one. We would go out to dinner and she would always pick up the bill. Sometimes we would have a few drinks together, though I knew my mother never drank on her own. At the LCBO we would look at the wine bottles and choose the one with the prettiest label. Neither of us knew anything about wine, so it came down to whether to get the red one with the fox or the white one with the monarch butterfly. We laughed at our innocence, and I remembered how, when I was little, my mother once made dandelion wine from the weeds she gathered from neighbours' lawns. She painted dreamy watercolour labels for the bottles, but she couldn't give the wine away.

One night, sitting with her on the living room futon, I asked her what she remembered about California in 1969. I had just read a book about the Source Family, a well-dressed cult that ran a health food restaurant on the Sunset Strip. Had she eaten there, I asked?

"I remember one time walking into a health food restaurant and thinking that the women who worked there looked so much healthier than me. I wasn't really very well back then."

Our conversation drifted to the recent American Thanksgiving party I had hosted. I explained that I hadn't invited a particular friend because I thought she would be put off by the smoking and drinking. I took a sip of wine and confessed that I was worried this friend might get uptight if someone tried to pass her a joint.

Joanna stiffened. "Promise me you don't do drugs!"

"Mom, relax, I'm just talking about pot. Honestly, pot seems a lot more harmless to me than alcohol," I said, swishing the wine in my glass and making a face at her. I was always making faces at my mother.

"No, I mean it. Promise me that you won't do drugs!" she repeated.

"Look, lots of people—people you like—smoke pot some-times," I argued, rattling off the name of a friend who had recently joined my mother and me for high tea.

"She isn't my daughter," my mother said. She paused, then switched gears. "Everything that's wrong with me is because of Allan."

Allan: her brother, my uncle. I became very still, the way you might around a skittish animal you want to catch.

"You let me spend the night at his house when I was a kid," I said.

"He was better by then," she told me. "And he would never . . . You were protected. I wasn't."

♥

BY THE TIME I was in my early twenties, I'd come to believe, to intuit, that my Uncle Al had sexually assaulted my mother. Over the years, she had dropped hints, but she would never discuss it openly. She would let a suggestion fall, then shut down my questions abruptly. "Damian, I don't want to talk about it."

I had always felt uncomfortable around Uncle Al. When he first said I looked like Brooke Shields, I was flattered. But the older I became, the more silently hostile I was in his presence. I didn't have language for why I acted this way, and I didn't talk to anyone about it. It had something to do with the way he looked at me—even though he was diffident around me, careful, apart. He never touched me. He avoided my eyes in a way that, in retrospect, reminds me of an awkward adolescent, though no one would have described him as boyish. For dinners at my grandparents' house, he would dress in short-sleeved button-downs, which he wore over undershirts, in a style not so different from my grandpa's. He had a short salt-and-pepper beard, a receding hairline, square-shaped glasses. We never had a one-to-one conversation, but as I grew older, I knew where he was in the room by an unpleasant physical sensation that flared through me; the hairs on my neck would rise, the inside of my ears buzzed. I felt a pressure against the bottom of my skull when my back was to him. By the time I was a teenager, I hated being anywhere near him.

This was before I suspected he had ever hurt my mother. He made my skin crawl, but from a distance. It was as if there were an invisible electric fence between us. He was polite, cautious, remote. Every interaction we had felt mediated, not by my mother or by my grandparents, but by this barrier. The older I became, the more conscious I was of sealing myself off from him.

Though I had heard my grandparents and my mother discuss his drinking problem, I only saw him on his best behaviour. My grandmother demanded the performance of normalcy from him and his wife and kids at family dinners; I think she felt that if we all behaved as if everything were okay, that would make it true. But the truth was that nothing was okay in his house—though I wouldn't know how bad it was there for years. In fact, I still don't know how bad it was. I know just enough to confirm it wasn't safe, for anyone. His oldest daughter told me that she once wrestled a gun out of his hands as it went off, leaving a bullet hole in the ceiling. My cousin Ann struggled with alcohol and drugs and spent years suffering in a violent relationship before dying of cervical cancer a few years ago. Her older brother was killed by lightning on a beach in Florida at the age of thirty.

My cousins didn't grow up in a safe home, but I did. I carried that safety with me, even when I was sleeping over with my cousins at his house. When I learned how unstable he was, I was angry with my mother. She insisted that I had never been in danger. I will never understand how she could have let me sleep there. In a way this seems delusional, tied to the family's deep denial, but it did feel as if there was a force field separating me from my uncle, a force field he could not cross.

My mother never had a protective force field around her.

When I was little, I thought Uncle Al said I looked like Brooke Shields only because I had prominent eyebrows like her. I had always remembered the first time I saw Brooke Shields when I was six years old, on that cover of *Seventeen* magazine, with the headline A MOVIE STAR AT 13 YEARS OLD. Her face—the glamour and strength and vulnerability of the way her eyes met the gaze of the camera—haunted me. I wanted to look like her, of course. But I saw something that was not fear, that was adjacent to fear, in her eyes, something raw and unsettled. It spooked me.

This was the year that the movie *Pretty Baby* was released. My mother didn't approve of *Pretty Baby*, a movie in which the then eleven-year-old Shields starred as the daughter of a prostitute growing up in a New Orleans Storyville brothel in the early twentieth century. Shields played Violet, and Susan Sarandon played Violet's mother, Hattie. In the scene where she leaves Violet behind in the brothel, Hattie reveals that her mother was a prostitute, that Hattie was also raised in a brothel. Hattie leaves Violet, but not before Violet's virginity is auctioned off. Shields stands on a table for this scene, wearing white lace and sausage curls, and the camera moves between Violet's face—her struggle to appear assured, her nerves showing—to the faces of the men assessing her, their mouths twitching at the edges. Everyone laughs when a deaf old man calls out "Fifty dollars" after the bidding has already tripled that figure. "Beautiful, Senator," someone chuckles good-naturedly—and so we know these are powerful men. Important men. "Remember, gentlemen," the madame calls out, "she is fresh as a baby's lips." After a fight nearly breaks out, Violet "goes" for four hundred dollars. In the movie poster, Shields sits on a porch holding a doll and wearing an impassive expression, bright mouth under a broad straw hat. Behind her, a thicket of palm fronds. "The image of an adult world through the eyes of a child" reads the copy beneath her feet.

This was Shields's first lead movie role, though she had modelled since she was a baby. Her first job had been an ad for white soap (the same brand my grandparents bought when my grandmother wasn't making her own soap with lye at the stove). When Brooke was ten years old, her mother arranged for her to be photographed by a man named Garry Gross. In a series of pictures that ran in a publication called *Sugar and Spice*, published by Playboy Press, she appears naked, wearing full makeup, posing in a claw-footed bathtub. In one photo her back is to the camera and her hair is pinned up with flowers; in another she blows soap bubbles, surrounded by lush houseplants. In the most shocking image, she stands in the tub, facing the camera, her arms outstretched, her skin shining. This is the image, appropriated by the artist Richard Prince, that the Tate Modern removed from an exhibit in 2009 after a warning from Scotland Yard.

The movie *The Blue Lagoon* came out when I was eight years old. On the film's poster, a permed Christopher Atkins reaches out with his left hand to tenderly hold Shields's face as the tanned teens gaze into each other's eyes, surrounded by palm fronds. (As in *Pretty Baby*, the plant stands in for exoticism and Edenic innocence.) The promotional copy for *The Blue Lagoon* celebrates the film's "sensual story of natural love." It goes on to say: "Two children, shipwrecked alone on a tropical island. Nature is kind. They thrive on the bounty of jungle and lagoon.

The boy grows tall. The girl beautiful. When their love happens, it is as beautiful as the sea, and as powerful." What the poster doesn't mention is that the two are cousins. I watched *The Blue Lagoon* with my cousin Ann, at her house. I watched the lovers swim under the turquoise water, aware that Shields's mother had insisted on a body double.

That same year, Richard Avedon filmed a series of Calvin Klein commercials with Shields. In one, she delivers a one-minute monologue about Darwin's theory of natural selection as she yanks on a pair of tight dark jeans, rolling onto her back to zip them before sitting up, unbuttoning the neck of her gold silk blouse on the phrase "selective mating," shaking out her long brown hair, then striking an improbable but compositionally pleasing pose, her arms on the ground, her legs akimbo and her ass in the air, as she lands on the line ". . . survival of the fittest." In another, she asks the camera, "Do you know what comes between me and my Calvins?" According to Shields, she never heard the double entendre in the question or her answer, "Nothing."

And then, in 1981, Brooke Shields starred in *Endless Love*, this time opposite Martin Hewitt, a dark-haired, then-unknown actor. The poster showed a close-up of their faces, their heads resting on linen-covered pillows. His eyes are closed, his mouth open and nearly on hers. Her eyes, heavy-lidded, are open. He is lost in the moment; she is observing it. In sleek lower case appear the words: "she is 15. he is 17. the love every parent fears."

There was a Brooke Shields doll, a Brooke Shields hairstyling mannequin head. There was also gossip and hand-wringing about her single-mother manager, who was portrayed in the press as an alcoholic who made bad choices for her daughter. And there were mixed messages from the actress herself. There was her anti-smoking campaign, which my mother told me Shields had to fight to do because of the controversy surrounding her public image. At my school library, the poster from this campaign showed Shields wearing a white jumpsuit that looked equal parts children's pyjamas and mechanic coveralls. It is zipped up to her neck. Cigarettes stick out of each ear, and above them the caption reads: "Smoking spoils your looks."

Brooke was really a good girl, my mother told me. A virgin, a student at Princeton. Brooke herself had written all about it in her autobiographical self-help book *On Your Own*, which my mother gave me for Christmas when I was in high school. I loved that book.

As an adult, I know Brooke Shields is not the trail of images created by men with cameras. I know the life of those images is not at all the same as the life of the young worker staring back at the lens. But I am also aware that part of the appeal of these images—part of what I sensed even as a young girl—lies in the ambiguity of her participation. She is a child being looked at, mostly by men. In the images, she appears to play along, and yet her innocence bleeds through. She appears pliable, unaware of the total effect of the image.

In every image of a beautiful girl performing the role of a beautiful woman, the viewer projects this tension onto the girl's face and body. This is especially true when the viewer feels that her face and her body don't match up. What do we even mean when adults name that tension *innocence*? The girl's incomplete awareness of her power is itself the source of that power. The source of her value. *She was a good girl.*

What does it mean that my uncle thought I looked like Brooke Shields? That I watched *The Blue Lagoon* in his house?

I was in danger. Yet I was protected; when she knew my uncle was drunk, Joanna drove to his house in the night and picked me up and took me home. My mother protected me.

But my mother was not protected.

I imagine Joanna at three years old, left alone with Allan when he was fourteen. I imagine she wanted to please him. I imagine he made her feel special. I imagine Joanna at three years old, four years old, five years old, six years old. Growing up in the same house I grew up in. The baby. Even when she was in her forties, everyone in the family called her "the baby."

When Joanna was six years old, her brother Allan turned seventeen and joined the navy. He left home and never lived in that house again. When she was eleven years old, Allan became a father. He had married a woman he'd met while based in Japan. Joanna was thrilled to be an aunt to her beautiful baby niece. She loved to babysit, she said; it was like playing with a real live doll. Joanna turned twelve, thirteen, fourteen. When Joanna was fifteen, Allan raped her.

Even now, it's so much easier for me to unpack the sexualizing of Brooke Shields, a child model and actress six and a half years my senior, than it is for me to process Joanna's ongoing molestation and violent rape at the hands of her brother—hands I remember, with their blistered blue anchors.

❦

FOR MY MOTHER, what happened to her body was inextricably linked to her brother's alcoholism and drug use. So, when she finally told me the truth about what had happened, she did so as a way of protecting me from the abyss of drugs and alcohol. Her truth was transactional: she gave me her most painful and shame-filled secret in exchange for the promise that I stop hurting myself. I imagine my uncle was drunk and high when he raped her. Maybe he got her high first. I'll never know.

All I know is what she told me: "Everything that's wrong with me is because of Allan."

Promise me you won't hurt yourself, she demanded. Promise you won't hurt me.

I promised. "But what happened with Allan?"

The strange thing is that I can't quite remember how she said it. Did she use the word *rape* first, or was it me who named it? She had told me years earlier, the afternoon she'd visited me at work in the clothing shop, that she had been raped at fifteen. But she would never tell me anything more about the situation. This night, finally, she said: "Yes, it was Allan." In fact, he had been molesting her since she was three years old. When he raped her, he would have been twenty-six, married, already the father of two.

My mother almost ran away from home, she told me, but a friend and her friend's sister intervened. Joanna was convinced by this young woman to tell her parents, my grandparents. Recently, since my mother no longer has the ability to talk about any of this, I connected with her high school friend and asked her what happened. Her friend replied in an email that she didn't know anything about it at all. But then she sent another message later, saying that, yes, she did remember. Joanna had come over to her house with her clothes dishevelled, distraught and very nervous and sad. That's all she could say, she told me.

That night in Toronto, Joanna told me that Allan had subsequently spent a year in some kind of mental health institution. She said with some bitterness that her brother Roger had picked Allan up when he was released. Until she was eighteen, she refused to be in the house when Allan visited my grandparents, and she left Michigan for California the year she turned nineteen.

"That's horrible," I said carefully and softly, when she finished speaking.

"Yeah, well, it wasn't a cakewalk," she said, flat defiance in her voice. She took another sip of wine. "I went to therapy and I'm okay. I'm fucked up with men, but other than that I'm pretty okay."

We sat unmoving for a moment on the couch, looking at each other. I was afraid to breathe.

"Promise me you won't write about this," she said.

IS FOR, IS FOR

*A is for absence, the ache of blank space I paste over with language.
B is for beauty, is for banishment. C is for candour. Not cruelty. Not
captivity. D is for descent, the deep dive, the desperate desire to document. E is for erasure, everything emptied of evidence. F is "for
you," forgetting. For form. For fear. G is for gratitude, guilt, grief
and the great goal to get it. H is for happiness, her heart holding out
for. I is for investigation, for the injuries of inquiry. J is for justice,
judgment and jury. K is for knife, the blade that creates the frame. L
is for love, the lamp I lift up. M is for making, for meaning, for
mixing my metaphors. N is for necessary. O is for the only option, for
or or or, our ongoing obligations. P is for pursuing patterns, for panic
and preservation. Q is for questing, for questions. R is for release, the
reach for the real. S is for seeking sense while slipping on switchbacks.
T is for tools, the tricks to trot out while tracking the trail. U is for
urgently untangling the undergrowth, for the ultimately unknowable.
V is for vanishing varnish. W is for words as welcome as water.*
     XYZ—examine your zigzags

PART II

ibis / icicle / idealism / identification
illegitimacy / I L L N E S S / illumination
illusion / illustration / image / imagination
imitation / impairment / imperative
imperfection / impermanence / impetuousness
implication / imposition / imposter / impression
imprint / imprisonment / improvisation / incest
incident / incoherence / individuation / infant
infection / infinity / infliction / infusion
ingenue / inheritance / inhibition / injury
inquiry / insider / insight / insouciance
inspiration / instruction / insulation / intelligence
intention / interference / interiority
internalization / interpretation / interrobang
interrogation / interruption / intervention
intimacy / intimidation / intrigue / intruder
intuition / invalidation / invasion / invective
investment / invisibility / inwardness / irritation
island / isolation / itch / ivy

When did her symptoms

How long do you think

Where did it start

JOANNA WAS QUIET as we sat and waited for the doctor. I did my best to make her feel okay about the appointment I'd made for her, but she ignored me. Her jaw was tight and her lips pressed into a thin line as she rubbed the base of her right thumb with the pad of her left. She'd relented and agreed to come, but she wasn't happy. When the doctor appeared and softly called her name, she followed him into his office and he shut the door.

While I waited, I spoke to the doctor's wife, who managed her husband's small practice. "His mother has Alzheimer's," she confided in me. "It's good what you're doing. I know it's hard, but you have to think about her safety. She could forget something on the stove and start a fire."

WHEN JOANNA FIRST moved to the Buffalo area to be closer to me, I had been frustrated with how she seemed incapable of managing her daily affairs without my help. I was irritated by her helplessness and I was impatient—short-tempered and resentful. My independence was everything to me. But as I visited her more often and we spent more time together, my annoyance turned to worry. I tried to talk to her about my concerns, but she froze up and blamed her lapses in memory and judgment on the fact that she had carpal tunnel syndrome and it was affecting her sleep.

> *I'm fine it's my thumb the pain keeps me up*
> *I'm just tired*
> *I'm just depressed*

The winter before I dragged her to a doctor, she had come to stay with Mike and me in Toronto over Christmas. It was there that she received the news that her house in Florida had sold after years on the market. But when she relayed this to me, she couldn't remember how much it had sold for. "Mom, it's important!" I yelled.

When, a few days later, her flight home was cancelled due to a snowstorm and rescheduled for the early hours of the following morning, she asked if I would still drop her off at the airport that night. She'd just stay up in the airport lounge, she said. We were in the living room, Joanna sitting beside me on the couch. She was fidgety, anxious. I couldn't tell if she didn't believe we would wake up in time, or if she didn't want to inconvenience us. We aren't dropping you off seven hours before your flight boards; that doesn't make any sense, Mike and I said. We'll wake early and take you in the morning. There's no reason for you to be at the airport all night. Exasperated, unable to convince us, she pulled a blanket over her head.

For weeks afterward, Mike would look at me and shake his head, reminding me, "She pulled a blanket. Over her head."

After her house in Florida sold, things moved quickly. Within months, she bought a small three-bedroom house in Lewiston, New York, minutes from the Canadian border, exactly where she'd dreamed of moving for years.

"If you have a baby, I can babysit," she told me. She'd been hoping I'd have a baby for years. When we lived in New York, she had often urged me to get pregnant, despite the fact that my life felt so unsettled. "You can give me the baby if you're not ready to be a mother," she'd joke. I think she was joking.

When I suggested to Mike, long before we knew she was sick, that my mother would probably be good with a baby, he replied, "She is a baby. The baby will be good with *her*."

One morning that spring, Joanna called me in a panic because the mover was on his way with all of her stuff and was demanding cash on arrival or he would throw it away. The following week she called me close to tears because she'd cancelled her cable and the man she'd talked to on the phone about it had told her he was taking thousands of dollars from her bank account. "He knows how," she told me, while I tried to reassure her this wasn't possible.

After she was finally set up in her new house, Mike and I took her to see Niagara Falls. She was amazed. "You know this is like fifteen minutes from your house, right? You can come here by yourself whenever you want," I told her. On another trip, we brought her to see the small but impressive collection of paintings at the Albright–Knox gallery. We stood before Marisol's *Baby*

Girl, a sculpture made out of rough-hewn wooden blocks. A tiny, doll-sized mother perched like a sparrow on the monstrous infant's giant thigh. Mike and I were, finally, trying to start a family and a psychic had recently assured me I'd have a child. "You have the shadow of a daughter on you," he told me. I just hope it's not my mother, I thought.

The summer before I dragged Joanna to the doctor, Mike played a show at the Art Park, near her new home. Joanna and I spent the afternoon together, talking about the young-adult science fiction novel she was writing. Then we walked to the park and danced in front of a stage surrounded by trees and the verdant green banks of the Niagara River. She shyly confessed to me that she had a crush on the architect a few doors down from her house but couldn't remember his name. Her neighbour across the street, an outgoing ninety-year-old widower, introduced himself to me. When Joanna wasn't listening, he told me, "I notice she sure seems to lose things a lot."

Six months after she bought the new house, Joanna lost her job, and I finally dragged her to the doctor. She had worked from home in Florida, and the company had originally agreed to let her continue to produce ads for their magazines remotely from upstate New York. Though they told Joanna they were merely restructuring, one of her colleagues had reached out to me even before the move, asking me to check in on my mother. "She's making mistakes on work she's been doing for fourteen years," she told me anxiously. They liked her there. When they let her go, Joanna's boss was gentle and promised her an excellent reference, but I knew something was seriously wrong. By then we'd learned that her brother in Florida had been living with early-onset Alzheimer's for several years, a fact he'd kept secret from the rest of the family for as long as possible. I'd begun to connect the dots. I spent my thirty-ninth birthday at my mother's home across the border, cleaning out her fridge—throwing out three or four opened jars of spaghetti sauce, half-eaten tins of salmon, old milk. I bought her string cheese, individual containers of yogurt, easy-to-heat single-serving soups. "We'll figure this out," I told her.

She never accepted her diagnosis, which the doctor had termed "moderate dementia." He warned me that she might decline quickly.

> *That doctor was a quack*
> *I was just so nervous*
> *I was just depressed*
> *Let me explain something to you*
> *I'm not senile*
> *My thumb hurts so bad I can't sleep*
> *How can I have dementia if I'm writing a book*

I talked to a friend of a friend, a lawyer in New York, who had gone through this with his father. He told me horror stories about what had gone wrong for their family. He advised me on what paperwork I needed to put in place immediately, how to make sure my mother always had forty dollars in cash, and how to get rid of her credit cards. "Disappear that shit," he warned me. I took notes on a stack of yellow Post-its as I sat in my brightly lit Toronto office. Before he hung up, he said, "Buckle up, sister." I wrote that down too.

❦

I DIDN'T THINK it was safe for Joanna to spend that winter alone, and luckily her sister invited her to stay down south for a few months. This was not a permanent solution, but it bought us some time. I reached out to the realtor who had just sold Joanna the house in New York and we put it back on the market. While we waited for it to sell, I paid a stranger to shovel the driveway. As I cleaned out Joanna's stuff, trying to figure out what to keep and what to let go, I found chequebooks with multiple attempts to write cheques for various bills—just "AT&T" written in the "pay to" line, but no more information— as well as other partially completed cheques, four or five of them, corresponding to the same, possibly still-unpaid bill. In every drawer I found an abandoned gratitude journal, the first few pages filled with the same nervous scrawl: *I am grateful for my wonderful daughter and son-in-law.* I threw all of these away.

I moved through that winter and spring in a constant state of gnawing anxiety. I couldn't function properly. At work events, people would ask, "How are you?" and I would say, "Not well." Then I'd dive into a long monologue about my mother's illness, and my helplessness.

"People just want to hear you say that you're fine when they ask that," Mike told me.

❦

OVER THE MOTHER'S DAY weekend, Mike and I realized a raccoon was living inside the walls of our enclosed back porch. We called a humane animal-removal service. A young guy with a goatee and coveralls inspected the house and confirmed that a raccoon was indeed living in the crawl space. He installed a one-way exit. The raccoon would be able to get out at night, but it would not be able to get back in.

The next day, a raccoon was desperately ripping roof tiles off the back extension, scratching and scratching at the blocked opening. It became clear that this was a mother raccoon, and she was going to rip the house to the ground if she had to in order to return to her babies. It was excruciating to watch. Her tail was spindly, her coat mangy. I kept thinking of Tom Waits singing that old nursery rhyme: "Hey ladybug, fly away home, your house is on fire and your children are alone."

I called the animal-removal guy again.

This time, he cut a hole in the ceiling of the back room and stuck his head up there. "Yep, I see them," he called down. He pulled on thick plastic gloves that reached to his elbows and disappeared into the crawl space. When he emerged, he was holding two squirming cubs by the scruff of their necks. They looked like stuffed animals. I had a strong urge to squeeze them tightly to my chest.

"They're so adorable," I said.

"Yeah, this one almost clawed my face off," the guy said, lifting the one in his right hand. Its tiny arms and legs wriggled in the air.

As the mother raccoon watched us from the roof of the garage, the guy lowered both baby raccoons into a large cardboard box with sides too tall for them to climb over on their own. He explained to me that the mother would retrieve them when she felt it was safe.

I stood at the side of the house, hidden, and waited. After a while I saw the mother slowly creep over to the box, then waddle over the side. She climbed the fence, carrying one baby carefully in her mouth, setting it down only when she reached the roof of the garage. Then she turned back around to fetch the other cub—but the first cub immediately followed her down. She looked back at the first one and then over at the second one still crying for her in the box. She brought the first cub back up to the garage roof and then again turned to fetch the second one. Again, the first one followed her.

Wait! Just wait there! She's coming back for you! Stay!

The first cub still trundled after the mother through the back-yard grass.

I went inside, unable to bear watching any longer.

❦

TO MARK MOTHER'S DAY, I had found an exhibit catalogue from a Marisol show online and sent it to my aunt's house, where Joanna was still staying. The catalogue, thin as it turned out to be, pleased her. Throughout those months when she was staying with extended family, we'd speak on the phone and email almost every day. She'd send me updates about her goings-on.

My mother emailed me early that summer:

> *In my new book the daughter kills the mother—she shoves her down the basement steps. Then she washes her and redresses her. She calls her ex-husband, who is going to come by plane to help her do something with this issue. Then she goes out and sleeps with a friend's son—he is an adult. This is before her ex-husband arrives. Then she goes back and the ex-husband*

arrives. It is quite a strange little book. Promise me you won't shove me down the stair.

❦

I'D WAITED UNTIL my late thirties to start trying for a baby. I'd waited to get my shit together. I'd waited to publish my first book of poems. I'd waited to finish a year at my fancy new job. I'd waited and waited because, though people told me otherwise, I believed I had all the time I needed. The time to start a family was always soon, just a bit of road ahead, five years, one year, next month. Maybe the month after next month. I'd waited for my ambivalence and anxiety to vanish. I'd waited until I sat in front of a doctor who had short brown hair and round wire-rimmed glasses, and who quickly sketched out a picture of my reproductive system: the cup of the uterus, the shrugging arms of the Fallopian tubes and the small bowls of the ovaries. My bowls, he explained to me in his soft Israeli accent, were empty.

The doctor's office was barely larger than a cubicle, but it had a door, and on his side of that door everything was white: white desk, white walls, white paper. A clean place to deliver bad news. An empty white chair beside me. Mike was on the other side of the country, finishing a west coast tour.

"We can keep trying, tracking your ovulation with blood tests and ultrasounds," the doctor told me as I stared at the blue ink. "We can do the intrauterine insemination and see what happens. But I don't recommend doing this for very long; it would be a waste of time and money. Is it possible you could get pregnant? Yes, but it is very unlikely. Maybe a four percent chance. You should start thinking about using an egg donor."

I felt as if he'd punched me in the gut.

"I'm under a lot of stress," I told him. I was shaking, my brain racing, scrambling. "Is it possible that this is affecting the test results?"

"You have a low ovarian reserve," he said carefully. He clearly regretted this part of his job, and he leaned into his professional compassion while gently but firmly pressing forward. He was nervous, and not unkind, but he wanted me to accept the situation so that we could look at solutions. "You will probably start menopause a bit earilier than average, probably not at forty but maybe at forty-five. It's hard to say."

"I'm sorry," he said.

I walked out of his office, past the aquarium and bank of massage chairs in the large waiting room filled with women like me, with couples who were all waiting for news, or for treatments that would lead to news. I held it together in the elevator, made it out to the street. I stood at the intersection of College and Bay, surrounded by medical buildings made of reflective glass. Then I called Mike. He answered, and I imagined him surrounded by the other guys in his band, trapped in the van, and I choked out the news to him. I stood in the middle of the flow of people, a self-contained storm on the sunny summer sidewalk, and wailed into the phone while the stream of the city parted around me.

"I love you. We'll keep trying," Mike said into the phone. "We'll figure it out."

The next day, my mother arrived to live with us.

labour / labyrinth / lace / lacquer / ladybug / lakes
lamb / lamentation / lance / landscape / lantern
lap / lasciviousness / latch / laughter / leaks / leap
leather / leaves / legacy / legends / legibility
lemonade / lemurs / leopard / letter / lettering
level / leviathan / levitation / lexicon / liability
liaison / liberal / libido / library / lies / lifeline
lightbulb / lightning / likeness / lilacs / lilies
limb / limbo / limits / line / link / lion / lip
liquidation / L I S T S / litany / literature
lizards / loadstar / lobe / location / lochia / lock
lollipop / looker / loon / loop / lore / lotion / love
loyalty / lucidity / luck / lust

MY MOTHER'S FAVOURITE MAGAZINE
WAS CALLED *PREVENTION*

Start fresh
27 days to a healthier, fitter, more energized you
Be your best self now
The answer is . . . yoga
15 power foods smart doctors eat (and love)
Good mood food
7 foods that should never cross your lips
Never diet again
Your body on coffee
Breathe easier with plants
Tap into your power
Banish brain fog
The beauty ingredient to avoid
Add two years to your life in 10 minutes
Can you smell when someone is sick?
Is your unwinding routine on repeat?
Is pain keeping you up all night?
Notice what feels good
Step 4: Find your happiness
"I am happy when _____"
Dream destinations: 13 trips to transform body and soul
Get out! Nature renews the mind
Your (gentle) wake-up call
The secret lives of American women
The pills that keep women afloat
Heaviest users: women 40 to 59
"I always felt like my hair was on fire"
Every mother counts
P.S. we're here for you
Goal: Reach your peak
Make this your best year ever

I USED TO joke that my mother would outlive us all.

Before arriving north in Canada to live with me and Mike, she had gone on a cruise with her sister, sailing from Miami to Freeport, Nassau and Great Stirrup Cay. In a souvenir photo of the two of them, Joanna is smiling in a coral-coloured T-shirt, her hands hanging in loose fists. On her shoulder I see the strap of the leaf-green leather purse that would later disappear, along with her wallet, her driver's licence, her passport.

After she was back with us, I wrote a poem (never finished) in which I referred to her as The Emergency. "Every morning The Emergency paces the kitchen floor waiting for me to wake up." Joanna woke up before dawn. Meanwhile, Mike and I were spending two to four hours per day at the fertility clinic before I headed into my office so that the doctors could monitor my monthly cycle with military precision. We slouched in the chairs ringing the aquarium and waited for ultrasounds, waited for blood tests—trying to get pregnant had become as demanding as a second job—and we kept receiving bad news. My ability to function professionally was shattered, and my colleagues let me know I was failing at follow-through. I met with an immigration lawyer about trying to move my mother to Canada, and he explained that, even if we were ultimately successful in our application, it would be years before Joanna would have access to any health care. I needed to find a safe place for her to live—knowing that the disease was only going to progress—but when I broached the subject of an assisted-living facility, she wept, begging me not to put her "in a home." We sat on the futon in the back room where she was sleeping, while I tried to explain how much freedom she would retain. "Please, Damian," she sobbed, "I'm not ready." It felt as if I was living inside a burning house, day after day, and nothing I did could extinguish the flames.

Sometimes Joanna would be stuck in a loop, a moment of endless present. It was not a state of grace, but one of terror and isolation. Trapped inside a continuous cycle of loss, she couldn't remember the events that had led her there and couldn't connect to what she might expect for the future, other than more and more fear. Mike did his best to try and make her laugh, calling her "Joanna Banana," and singing silly songs for her. He cooked her lunch every day when I was at work, paying attention to her new favourite things to eat (hot dogs and pizza). Sometimes she'd smile, but other times she'd accuse us of plotting against her.

In a lucid moment, she sent me an email from inside the house: *It is hard for me to have this illness and I don't mean to take it out on you. I just feel like I have lost everything.*

Once, my mother and I were walking together past the Centre for Addiction and Mental Health, not far from my house, and we came across a woman who was clearly, publicly suffering. A stone wall runs along the east side of the health centre grounds— the last section of a barrier built in the nineteenth century when this had been the site of the Provincial Lunatic Asylum. This is where we passed the woman, whose face was contorted with a pain that was difficult to witness. The woman shouted an incoherent stream of invective, although there didn't seem to be a fixed target for her rage. Joanna and I walked on. After a few beats, my mother turned to me, her face animated by her own anger. "When I get like that," she said, "just shoot me."

That summer, Mike and I drove out to the country to take Joanna to a place called Nova's Ark, an animal sanctuary run by a woman who had worked as a special education teacher. All of the animals had been rescued from danger in one way or another. While we walked the grounds, Mike took short videos on his phone of my mother and me with various creatures: a fawn, a wombat, a pair of macaw parrots. In one video, my mother and I are squealing in front of a large fenced-in enclosure where the three lemurs lived. My mother is wearing a navy-and-white-striped long-sleeved shirt and jeans. I'm wearing a second-hand wine-coloured cotton sundress. We kneel together, our backs to the camera, mesmerized by one of the lemurs, who is dragging around his pet cat like a big fluffy stuffie. The cat, which had nearly died after being run over by a car before being nursed back to health at the sanctuary, deferred completely to the lemur, even though she was twice its size. Joanna and I lean into each other and laugh as we watch them play.

Joanna loved animals. I noticed when she returned from staying with her sister, where she had seen another doctor, who had confirmed her dementia diagnosis, that she had been writing out animal names in her notebooks, over and over. I asked her about it and she explained, a little evasively, that she was memorizing a list of more than 150 different animals. Sitting at her laptop, she googled "mandrill monkey" and took notes from the Wikipedia entry that popped up. Then she googled "dance of the blue-footed booby" and showed me a video of the male bird's mating display. "I love this, I love this!" she cried, pointing and laughing as the brilliant-blue feet lifted slowly up and down on a Galapagos rock. On her screen, the male raised his head, long beak pointing to the sky, pupils dilating, and stretched his black-and-white-feathered wings out wide, still rhythmically lifting his feet, back and forth, marching in place. We watched as the female turned her head away and preened her own feathers, apparently unimpressed. I smiled.

Later, my mother admitted that she had planned to take the lists back to show the doctor she'd seen when she was staying with her sister, as documentation to prove she didn't really have dementia. Her sister shut that down. "She told me he wouldn't want to see them," my mother told me sadly. But she didn't stop making the lists. Even after she moved into an assisted-living residence in Buffalo, she kept filling notebooks and sketchbooks with these numbered lists of animal names. She wrote the lists inside the covers of the books she borrowed from the facility's common room, inside the covers of her own books and across every scrap of paper she found.

❧

BEFORE SHE DIED, Mike's grandmother had lived in a lovely facility in Toronto that I was using as a model for what might be right for my mother. I learned a new vocabulary: "assisted-living facilities" offered more support than an apartment but more creature comforts and opportunities for independence than a nursing home. Some felt like pumped-up condos for the elderly, featuring amenities such as movie rooms with padded theatre seats that ran old films twenty-four hours a day, free frozen yogurt or popcorn dispensers, beauty parlours. Some felt more like hospitals with slightly better lighting and more bad art. I wanted to preserve as much of my mother's autonomy as possible, for as long as possible, and I chose the wrong place as a result. If I had a time machine. You learn all the most important lessons about how these systems work in the wrong order. We cashed out all of my mother's savings and, because she always lived frugally and was responsible about her money, there was enough to pay for two years at a nice facility. Many of the nice facilities had an informal policy that after a resident drained all of their private financial resources and transitioned to Medicaid, the facility would keep the resident in their care. A lawyer I'd hired to help with the legal paperwork had advised me to select a place like this, warning me that if we had to move my mother when she was already on Medicaid, the options would be limited to places "you'd never want a loved one to live."

I did a lot of research and found an assisted-living residence that was part of a larger, linked network of care facilities, including nursing homes, that I believed would provide her with advancing levels of care as her needs escalated. The company had a good reputation, and the location I settled on was next door to a public library. There was a farmers' market every Saturday in the summer just on the other side of their parking lot. She could walk to her bank, to dollar stores and bookstores and cafés. I imagined her visiting the nearby animal shelter and petting the kitties. She would live in a small studio apartment with her own bathroom and kitchenette but take all her meals in the main dining room with the other residents. Community, I thought, would do her good. A shiny black piano stood in the corner of the carpeted lobby, and I thought maybe she would play it. She had not liked giving up the family piano.

Joanna moved into the facility in mid-December. "An early Christmas present for you!" said the eldercare counsellor we hired to help us fill out forms. "Eldercare counsellor": a job I'd never known existed.

For a while, I could breathe again. By February, I was pregnant. A miracle. I couldn't face the sterile clinical procedures that month, and we ended up getting lucky the old-fashioned way. The head of the clinic, a warm man with a full white beard, congratulated me when he heard this and said, with a smile, "I didn't know that worked." He showed me, during an early ultrasound, a tiny winking light on the screen. "Look at that, a heartbeat," he said. "Splendid!"

Mike and I were ecstatic.

❧

AT FIRST, JOANNA adapted well to the assisted-living facility. Unlike most of the other residents, my mother hadn't grown up in the area. A lot of her fellow residents, meanwhile, had attended prom in the very room where meals were served, as the building had been a Masonic Temple. The dining room's ceiling was painted deep blue, with gold stars scattered across it. That ceiling gave me a faintly hopeful feeling.

Most of the people who lived in this place were eighty or older. My mother befriended a 103-year-old woman named Millie. She would knock on Millie's door and walk her to the dining room for every meal. "They are two peas in a pod," said the facility's administrator, a friendly man who ended many of our conversations with the promise to pray for us. "The oldest and the youngest residents we have. I call them our odd couple," he chuckled.

In the beginning Joanna flourished there. Or, if not exactly flourished, she did her best. She helped Millie and other older residents by walking them to meals. She would visit a retired priest in his room and do his dishes. She made her bed every morning, she dressed neatly. She decorated her windowsills with seashells and agates and small crystals arranged in patterns. She propped up an illustration with a quote by Emerson that she liked next to a rabbit figurine.

Millie died six months after my mother moved into the facility. Soon, Joanna stopped letting the aides do her laundry each week. She started referring to her fellow residents as "the other inmates." The social worker at the facility called me. She was concerned about Joanna, who had developed a habit of walking the halls at a fast pace. One day she passed out. After I hung up, I called my mother on her cellphone.

"I'm not like everyone else here," she told me. "They're all going to die."

She had realized that all of her attachments would end in grief there. She wanted to leave, she said. She wanted to get a small apartment, and a cat. "I hate not having a cat."

As I tried to calm her down, she grew angrier and angrier with me. "THERE'S NOTHING WRONG WITH ME!" she shouted, and then she was gone.

❦

IN AUGUST, WHEN I was seven months pregnant, the administrator who liked to pray for us called me at work. Joanna had withdrawn all of her money from the bank and was hiding the cashier's cheque. She was convinced I was stealing her money.

I called my mother and tried to talk to her.

"You need to grow up and get a job," she yelled at me.

"Mom," I yelled back, "I have a job! I have a really stressful job! I am at my job right now!"

She hung up.

Shortly after that, my mother became fixated on a woman who worked as an aide in the building. "She comes into my room at night and tries to hook me up to a drug drip," she told me. "She is stealing my toilet paper."

Then my mother packed up her things and announced she was going back to Florida. She threw out boxes of stuff, including a seemingly endless supply of the book *Harold and the Purple Crayon*. She barricaded her door with a wooden side table my grandfather had made. "My daddy made this to protect me," she told me.

My mother felt vulnerable, aware that the residence's staff had access to her room at all times of the day and night. There was no way to lock the door.

"Everyone in this place has a key," she told me.

WHEN MY MOTHER WAS DIAGNOSED WITH DEMENTIA, SHE TRIED TO MEMORIZE MORE THAN 150 ANIMAL NAMES

white-spotted skunk, black-footed ferret
mandrill monkey, howler monkey
ocelot, Arctic hare, grey mouse lemur
animals racing across the surface of sketchbooks
animals filling journals, names inserted inside borrowed novels
armadillo, gazelle, porcupine
sometimes stray notes attached: *acrobat*
Manx cat—appeared naturally 300 years ago
reputation for ferocity
she tapped into her computer and showed me
the slow sweet dance of the blue-footed booby
laughing laughing "Isn't he a scream?"
as I emptied each drawer, I found new lists
lists torn from notebooks, folded and crammed
lists inside the jacket covers of self-help classics
the 7 habits of highly effective
buffalo, moose, ostrich, bloodhound, lamb
names scrawled in pen across two pillowcases
animals running all night through her dreams

zap / zeal / zebra / zenith / zephyr / zest
zigzag / zilch / zinc / zip / zit / zodiac
zombie / Z O O

122. ARDVARK 123. ~~Osolot~~.
123. GRAY FOX 124. DINGO
125. prairy Dogs 126. African wild cats
   TOWNS
127. AFRICAN wild dogs.

THE

SEVEN

SPIRITUAL

LAWS

OF

SUCCESS

128. Snowshoe Hare 129. white Rat
130. Giant Anteater 131. Kinkajou
132. Ape ~~13~~ 133. ALPACA
134. BOAR 135. Civet 136. Cougar
137. ~~Elk~~ ELK 138. Eland ~~39~~.
139. Ground Hog 140. white Rat
141. Caraibu or Rain deer
142. Gi

North American River Otter
Curacao Vampire Bat
Leopard Gecko

Vampire Bat
feeds
on mammals
Blood Animals
& Humans

Common Bat

Bulargu Whale = White Whale

Ocelot = Ocelot - dappled fur
Couguar = Couguar

Tarantula —   hairy Arachnids

Cicada = widely
            Apart
AMAZON HORNED Frog

136. White Handed Gibbon
137. Moles sence of smell 138. Howeler Monkey

139. YAK 140. Shaggy Hair - Matted
140. Zebra   ] under coat
141. Kowala Bear   ┌ INSOLATED to
     Remain in Pouch │ Against
     At Least 6 Mounths│   COLD
                       └

                 fox
142. Gray Wolves
143. Reses Monkeys 144. Dormouse
144. Przewalskies Wild Horse
146. African Austrailian Ibis
148. African Sacred Ibis,
147. Tasmainian Devel 149. Canadian
148. American Red Squirrel ┌ LYNX
149. Rebel Mongoose - Slim - Animals
                       Coarse Speckeled
150. Water Buffolo   Hair
151. Siaberian Tiger 152. Kowala
                              Bear
153. Zebra 154. Mongoose
155. Gorilla 155.

49

8 → This one for sure!

8 Bears - 1. American Black Bear 2 Sloth Bear

3. Kowala Bear 4 Pollar Bears 5. Alasican Brow Bean

6. Kodiak Bear 7. Gizzley Bear & Black speckled

Foxes: 9. Bateared Fox 10 Fennic fox "Little ₂₂ Bear
"Little Bear 11 Flying Fox 12. Artic Fox

Armadillo's 13 Pink fairy Armadillo 14 Hairy Armadillo

15. Giant Armadillo Kangaroo's 16 Matschie's
Tree Kangaroo

17. Large Red Kangaroo 18. Eastern Grey Kangaroo

19. Yellow footed Rock Wallche 20 Rock Wallaby Kangate
Brush tailed Rock
20 Musky Rat Kangaroo - Smallest. Wallabie

Leopard 22 Snow leopard 23 Cloud Leopard 24 Leopard Lynx

24 American Bison 25. American Buffolow

Jackal's 26 Golden Jackal 27 Black Backed Jackal
Jackal
28. Side striped Jackal 29. African Elephant

Cats 12
30. Egyiphian Mou 31. Siamese 32 Tonka

33. Abyasinnian 34. Burmese 35. Bombay

36. American Bobtail 37. Forest cat 41 Main Coon
short
38 Don Spkynx cat 39 Ragamuffin 40 Munchkin

41 Main Coon Dogs 42 Akita 43 Jack Russel

9 Dogs 44 Welsh terrier 45 Welsh Springer Spaniel

46 American Bull dog 47 Basset Hound 48 Yorkie

49. Fox Terrier 50 Whippet more →

✗ Yes this is the one/ 36.

HYMLAYON

#1. Giant Panda Bear #2 Redpanda SMALL

#3. Bengal tiger & Bengal tiger white

#5 & FENNIC FOX small BIG EARED fox

#6 Galupogus tortist Giant

#7. Asian Black Bear - #8 SUN BEAR moon Bear of tibet

#8. Shoth Bear - SLOPPY (worngspla) #9 Pollar Bear

#10 - Alaskar BROWN Bear #11 Kowala Bear

#12 MANDRIL MONKey old world #13. Rhinosourus

#14 Rhinoscrus white #15 badgers

#16. MATSHIE'S TREE KANGAROO Australier Rainforest

#17 DwarfLeopard ocelote #18 white tailed deer

#19. NORWAY Rat - 3rd BROWN Rat 27 mule

#20 Rat PINKeyed white Rat 24 Gibben

#22. Bob Cat #23 Giraffe 28 Mercat

#25 western Low Land Gorila

#29 29. SpottED Hyena 30 LAMA

#30 Timber Wolf #31 Zebra

#32 Mountuin Goat 33 ASIAN Lions

#34 BLACK Panther 36. Moose

#35 American BUFFOLO 37. ELK

Egyptian Mbo - Siamese
Cats

175. TONKA - Cat - Forest cats
176 Burmese cats -
177 Abysinian cats -
178 short Haired cats
179 Long Haired cats
180 MAIN COON cat
181 Bombay cat
182 Forest cat
183 DON Sphy NX cat
184
185
186
187
188
189
190
191
1921

PRAYER Before Birth

Louis MacNeice

I AM NOT yet born; O hear me.
Let not the blood sucking bat or the RAT
OR the stoat or the
clubfooted ghoul come near me.

I AM NOT yet born; console me.
I fear that the human RACE MAY with
TALL walls WALL me,
With strong drugs me, with dope
me, with wise Lies Lur me,
ON black racks rack me, in
blood-bad

babble / B A B Y / background / backslide
baffle / balance / ballad / balm / band / bane
banishment / bankruptcy / banks / barrage
barricade / barrier / base / basement / basin
bath / battle / beach / beam / bear / beast / beat
beauty / bed / bedlam / beetle / behaviour / belief
belittlement / bell / belligerence / belly
belongings / beloved / bend / beneficiary
benevolence / betrayal / bewitchment / beyond
bind / biography / biology / birds / bitterness
blame / blankness / bleakness / blessing / blight
blinders / bloat / blocks / bloom / blossom / blot
blur / body / bohemian / bolt / bond / bones
books / boot / booze / boundaries / boyfriends
brain / bramble / bread / breath / brief
brightness / brilliance / broadcast / brokenness
brother / brow / bruise / brunette / brush
bubble / buckle / buffalo / bugaboo / bugbear
bugler / builder / bumblebee / bungalow
burden / bureaucracy / burrow / butterfly
button / buzz / bye-bye

FOR YEARS, JOANNA had a recurring dream that she had suddenly found herself with a baby in her arms and had no idea what to do with it. Stuck without a crib, she opens a dresser drawer and lays the baby down on a pile of soft clothes. The baby, she thinks, will sleep comfortably there until she finds a better solution. Then she absent-mindedly shuts the drawer with the baby inside it and leaves the house. She forgets about the baby for a while, and the dream continues in other directions. Then suddenly, with a flash of panic, she remembers. The baby! She has to get back to the baby!

This dream never reached a resolution; it ended inside the lightning bolt of fear and anxiety: she has abandoned her baby; her baby is in great danger. We discussed the dream one time, when she still lived in Michigan and I was visiting her. I suggested perhaps the baby represented the fact that she hadn't felt prepared to become a mother. No, she said.

"The baby in my dream isn't you," she corrected me. "The baby is me."

When I was seven months pregnant, my mother had a psychotic break. Not only did she drain her bank account and hide the cashier's cheque for $57,110.15 in her closet; not only did her wallet and passport disappear, permanently; not only did she tell the staff at the assisted-living facility and the women who worked at the bank that I was trying to steal her money, she also told them I wasn't really pregnant. There's no baby, she insisted. When I waddled into Bank of America to redeposit the money so that Mike and I could keep covering the cost of her care, the teller said, "She told us that you were taking her money to drink and do drugs. I told her you were just paying her bills."

I thanked the woman, though I felt she was eyeing me a little suspiciously.

"She said you're not really pregnant," the woman continued.

"Well, I am," I said, my hands opening out over my giant belly.

"She said you poisoned her," the woman said in a lower tone.

"I didn't," I whispered back.

ALL THE MESSAGES MY MOTHER LEFT
THAT I WROTE DOWN AND LATER ERASED

Hi Damian? Did you call me? You or Mike? . . . [inaudible] . . . Damian? . . . Mike? . . . She's not there . . . Hello? Damian? . . . Damian?

Hey there, I thought that you had called at some point, I didn't realize it. If you need to, call me back in a little while, okay?

Hey sweetheart, I didn't know you called and then I just tried to get you and if you're busy don't worry about it and you know you can come see me any time you want, bye-bye.

Hi Damian, this is your mama and I just wanted to see how you were doing okay? Bye-bye.

Hi Damy, this is your mother and I yelled at the man who yelled at—who wasn't nice to you so—and I made him clear on what was really wrong in the world, so um I want you to be better and I want you to feel better and when you get the chance maybe we could chat or something okay? I love you.

Hi this is your mommy and I yelled at that man and told him not to do that again so you don't have to worry about that. I love you and I hope you're not unhappy okay? Bye-bye.

Hey there it's just me and I'm just calling to see how you're doing. Though I'm seeing everyone around and so I'll talk to you later.

Hey it's me, your mother, and I need a little help from you, um, I have someone who I came home from lunch and . . . you know . . . whatever it is . . . and . . . she was coming to . . . somebody who's not supposed to be in here and she and her friend are trying to steal in and so if she . . . you can tell the staff they're here, you'll have to wait till a little bit earlier, later, because they won't be open, and let them know that she's been doing that so that I can get out of the room again? Thank you.

Ouch . . . Hey there it's me. Hey I have a little, a couple of little things for your son that I was going to send to you and I don't know if you want me to or not . . . it's a cute little car . . . little . . . you know it looks like a cat-thing and on top of it is a little . . . red bird, and it's real cute and the other one is [inaudible] and if you want them I'll send them to you and if not [inaudible]. Thank you.

Hi and it's just me and I'm just calling to see how you're doing, okay? Bye-bye.

Hey this is your mother and I know I called and left a message that I would make whatever you wanted and I would make it as nice as possible for you and you're mad at me that I wasn't able to bring . . . to do it. If you'd come in I could [inaudible] I couldn't [inaudible]. So try to get over it and—and realize that I have to get out of here tomorrow. I love you, I'm sorry that—that's it, I promise that I'll do everything I can to make, make—make things come in money for you okay? I'll do everything I can to do that. If you just give me a shot. Alright? Bye-bye.

Hey Damian? Are you there? Are you there Damian? Um, I lost . . . I can't get you back here, can you call me up? [inaudible]

Damian I have no money to give you. I offered you . . .
that's all the stuff I have. I don't have anything else.
There was no money. I gave you [inaudible] That was a
long time ago [inaudible]. Please try to get your name
as a nice person back in this world.

Hi I realize you're very, the kind of person who thinks
everything is going to happen the way you want it
to . . . It doesn't. I didn't do anything . . . I didn't have
anything, I still don't have anything, and you're still
trying to get it from me and you're hurting me and
you're hurting yourself, so stop it.

Damian I do not have any money whatsoever and you
have this woman and I don't need her here, there's no
reason for it, there's absolutely no reason for you to
do that and now I don't have any money whatsoever.
So grow up!

Hey I got your flowers, they're beautiful, thank you so
much! Bye-bye.

Damian why do you keep sending these people to me,
I have no money, absolutely no money what—at all. I
know ███ said something but she lied. She likes lying
because it makes it harder for me . . . to . . . [inaudible].
I need you, I don't . . . need a thing from you. All I had was
what I had and I don't have anything left [inaudible].

Hey there it's me, I need to know why you're doing this
with these people. I don't have any money for anyone,
I only have like five—five things that I could even give
them. Now I can't do anything with this. I don't know
why you're upset but I'm pretty sure ████ was
involved. ████ is an evil person and she tells a lot of

lies. So you know, come back to the fold. Be my friend again and my daughter okay? Bye-bye.

Hey there, um, I wish I could do something for you, but I can't, but uh, you need to get a job and work and then you won't have any problems. [inaudible] You really have to if you're going to have anything okay? I'm sorry about it but [inaudible]. Okay, bye-bye.

When I die you're going to prison. Forever.

Hey there it's me and I just wanted to see how you were doing and everything was going alright and . . . I don't have as much . . . Anyway, I'm hoping . . . [inaudible]. Bye-bye.

Hey this is your mother and I just wanted to tell you that I love you and I'm hoping you're having a nice day and I'll talk to you later okay? Bye-bye.

Honey it's just me and I just need to hear your voice and you're alright. Alright? It's just frightening me. Okay? Bye-bye.

Hey there it's me and right now nothing's going wrong but I'm wondering if you'd do me a favour and give me the number of um . . . the . . . people who come in and save you. Here, in this particular place where I am. I don't think anything's going to happen but I like to be prepared. Okay? Thank you sweetheart I love you.

Hey it's me, I was wondering could you . . . call Buffalo, where I am, and get the names of who I could call if something went wrong? Okay? Thank you sweetie.

Honey I don't want you to come today. I love you but I can't have you come. This woman . . . I . . . at any rate . . . don't come today alright? Maybe next week? Or whenever it's convenient after that. I'm sorry, it's just that something's come up that's going to make it really difficult and I just don't want to get into any problems, alright? I love you, please forgive me, and have a nice time, okay?

Hey there I just wanted to know that you're alright and everything's going well. This is your mama. Okay? When you get a chance call me. Bye-bye.

This is me and I've accepted the fact that I'm not going anywhere so you don't need to bother coming here. Okay? Bye-bye.

Hey there this is your mama and I wondered if you're back and okay, okay?

I just wanted to tell you that you know when you have that baby that the pain is significantly less than when you poisoned me so I should think you shouldn't have any trouble. Okay? Bye-bye.

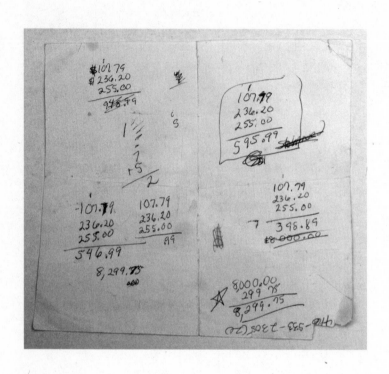

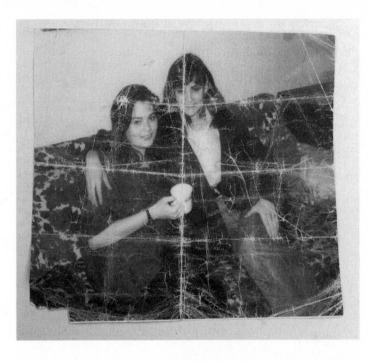

**COLOUR PRINTOUT OF A PHOTO TAKEN
BEFORE I MOVED TO ENGLAND IN 1993**

*Joanna had folded and unfolded this photocopy many
times. On the back she had calculated how much
money she believed I'd stolen from her account while
she was in an assisted living facility.*

nacre / nadir / naiad / naiveté / nakedness

N A M E S / naps / narcissus / narcosis

narration / narrowness / nastiness / nasturtium

nativity / nature / naught / naughtiness

nausea / navel / navigation / neatness

nebulousness / necessity / necklace / nectar

neediness / needle / negation / negativity

neglect / negligee / negligence / neighbour

neophyte / nephew / nereid / nerves

nervousness / nest / net / nettle / network

neurologist / neuromodulation / neutral

newspaper / next / niceness / nickname

nicotine / niece / nightgown / nightlight

nightmare / nipple / nobility / node

noiselessness / noncommitment / nonsense / nook

noose / normalization / north / nostalgia

notebooks / nothingness / notice / notoriety

nouns / nourishment / novel / novice / nowhere

nuance / numbers / numbness / nuptials / nurse

nurture / nutrition / nymphet

NAMES ARE HOW we hold on to things. One of the first clues for me that Joanna was suffering cognitive decline was how often she was forgetting words, especially nouns. Language loss is common with various forms of dementia; the language centre in the brain breaks down. As my mother misplaced the names for things, the things themselves slipped out of her hands.

I was nine months pregnant, and only a few hours before my water broke, a small blue teapot that had belonged to Mike's grandmother split apart and slipped out of my own hands. I already knew I was carrying a boy. ("That's good," Joanna had said when I shared this news with her three months into my pregnancy. "Girls can be rivals for Daddy's attention." I can't imagine my mother saying something like this before her illness; I wonder, though, now, if she still might have thought it.) Mike and I had already chosen the name Levi. I liked it because I'd read that it means "joined in harmony" in Hebrew. I held my belly and hummed.

Later, after the birth, the woman who worked the reception desk at the assisted-living facility told me what had happened when she'd asked Joanna for her new grandson's name. My mother had immediately gone upstairs to her room and checked the paper where she'd written the name down. When she returned, she said proudly, "It's Levi. The baby's name is Levi."

When Levi was born, my mother forgave me for all my crimes, real and imagined.

❧

WHEN JOANNA HAD lived with us in Toronto, before entering assisted living in Buffalo, I had brought her with me to a poetry event where I had been invited to read. This was the first time she'd seen me read my own work since I was in university.

I read a poem with the line "I can't go on like this, always a Damian." A week later, a journal that had published a few of my poems, including that one, arrived in the mail. My mother and I sat together at the kitchen table, and I watched as she read the words with pleasure, laughing at the jokes, smiling. But when she reached that line, her mouth twitched.

"I'm sorry you don't like your name," she said.

"No, Mom, that's not what that line means. I'm glad you named me Damian," I said. "Really."

❧

PEOPLE ALWAYS ASK, "Does your mother know who you are?"

One day an aide asked her, "Who's this, Joanna?"—pointing to me—and my mother said, "This is someone who came to talk to my sister."

"Your sister? I thought she was your daughter," the aide said.

My mother looked around the room, nodding, while I held her hand.

For the first time, I thought to ask her if she knew my name.

"No," she said.

"It's Damian," I told her.

"You're playing games with me," she said, giving me a look that said, *enough jokes*.

I laughed. "You're the one who named me. You know I'm your daughter, right?"

"Yeah, yeah," she said, looking across the room.

It was spring. I was staying in Buffalo by myself, visiting my mother every day. Every day she was incrementally happier to see me.

One night at dinner, a nurse asked the question again. "Who is this, Joanna?"

"She's a friend."

"I'm your daughter," I said, and kissed her.

"You two look so much alike," the nurse said.

The day after that, another nurse asked Joanna who I was.

"She's my daw—daughter," my mother said. As she paused in the middle of the word, I could see her working to find the second half of it.

"What's her name?" asked the nurse.

"Dam-innn," my mother mumbled. I squeezed her hand.

I was returning to Toronto the next day. I told my mother I

had to go home and take care of my son—*Levi*—and tears welled in her eyes. We stood in the hallway, and I held her. I wish I didn't have to leave, I told her. I'll be back soon, I told her. We stood there holding each other for what felt like a long time before I finally pulled away.

That was the last time I heard her say my name.

kaleidoscope / karma / keepsake / kettle
keyboard / keyhole / key-liner / K E Y S / kicker
kid / kin / kindergarten / kindling / kindness
kindred / kineticism / kingdom / kismet / kiss
kitchens / kitten / knack / knave / knell / knife
knock / knowledge

I get paid in two weeks so I
    can send you money I arranged
        transportation for a couple dollars a month
            I've limited myself to 25 cents a day (coffee)
            Except for one day a week 45 cents

It will cost me $9.86 to work a month I will spend
    a grand total of $32 a month for store items
        Clothing I'm too fat and tall for mine
            Stockings makeup perfume shoes
            Gifts (for you darling)

$41.86 a month on doctors dentists and you darling
    $375 in three months $725 in six months
        I could pay for us both to go to Europe
            aren't I awfully clever for being so dumb

IT WAS AFTER Levi was born that my father sent me the box containing all the letters my mother and I had ever sent him. Along with the letters my mother had written to my father during my childhood, sending him updates about my progress at school or swimming, or how tall I'd grown, and along with the later letters I'd sent thanking him for birthday and Christmas cheques, I found a letter my mother had written my father in 1971, when she was pregnant with me. She had been living with her parents in Michigan, working part-time at a department store, and was desperate for him to come see her. It's heartbreaking to read—she sounds delusional, unstable and passionately in love.

Around this same time, when I visited Joanna, she would share stories with me I'd never heard her tell before. Of course, now I had no way of knowing if they were true or not. One day, she began talking about what it had been like to live in California. It wasn't very nice, she said. The houses were too close together.

She talked about her ex-husband, accidentally calling him Mike one time. I corrected her gently. She paused, and then repeated the name I had just given her, in the voice of a student lacking confidence in the answer. At the time, I assumed she had confused her husband's name with my own husband's name. But there's another possibility. Mike was also the name of her husband's friend, the one who had lived with them for a while in California—the one she told me she had thought she was in love with for a while. This was a period when she time-travelled, the past surfacing in surprising new ways.

After a while, her memories took a dark turn. She began to tell complicated stories about her ex's father, who she said had "beat the shit" out of her ex when he was young. Her ex had been beaten so severely, she explained, that he would never be able to have children. "I didn't know that," she said to me, "and one day I said to him, oh maybe we'll have a baby, and he got so angry. He thought I must be having an affair, since he couldn't get me pregnant, and he beat the shit out of me."

"That's terrible," I told her. "I'm so sorry."

❦

JOANNA'S STATUS AT the facility was precarious. After she had moved in, the entire network of linked facilities had been sold to a large company based downstate, and the staff kept changing. As her illness progressed and she continued to behave erratically, a new administrator labelled her an "inappropriate resident" and an "elopement risk." Another resident had slipped out in the middle of the night and died of exposure over the winter and my mother, who had once announced that no one liked her and she was leaving, was seen as a legal liability. But the company wouldn't move her to one of their facilities with a locked memory-care unit or into one of their several nursing homes. We received an eviction notice, which I'd successfully staved off, temporarily at least, with the help of an eldercare lawyer and a small group of advocates I'd found online. I became friendly with a woman who worked at the Department of Health. I lived in fear of incoming phone calls from the Buffalo area code.

If I had a time machine.

When my mother's bank account balance fell below the regulated threshold, we applied for Medicaid. After she was approved due to her inability to live safely on her own, the facility moved her into a smaller room, and we purged more of her things. I sat on the floor with her, going through photo albums, and threw away so many pictures of people she no longer recognized.

She had been on Seroquel, a powerful antipsychotic, for over a year, and she was no longer allowed out of the building. Her physical health deteriorated. The lack of exercise and the institutional food had contributed to her gaining more than fifty pounds in a few months. She still looked younger than she was, her hair dark and shiny, but her skin had a waxy sheen, and her eyes lacked light.

She started to tell me stories I'd never heard before, and I didn't know which ones were real and which ones were not. One day, I was alone with my mother in the small shared lounge outside her new room, and she told me a story about living with my father and me in Detroit when I was an infant. In this story she was alone in the apartment with a man, not my father. A stranger? A neighbour? A friend? Her stories lacked important details. She said that the man told her, "Don't worry about the baby, put the baby in the crib. Come into the other room with me, the baby is fine." She said that she did what he told her to do.

"Then he raped me," she said. "Isn't that terrible?"

I was horrified and told her so.

"And last week," she said quickly, "this man came into my room here and he told me—he said, go over there—" She waved her hand in the direction of her bedroom, which was sandwiched between two other women's rooms. "And then he raped me. Isn't that terrible?"

Whenever my mother spoke of violence during this period, real or imagined, her tone did not match the content of her speech. Her delivery was the same as how she once might have told me a story about going to the freezer and realizing the ice cream she had been planning to eat for dessert was missing. "Isn't that terrible?"

Another day, she told me that her brother Allan had been violently sexually assaulted when he was thirteen years old, during a few months when all four of the kids were living with their paternal grandmother in a small town in Pennsylvania. This town was so small that no one bothered to number the houses for another thirty years. It was there, according to my mother, that Allan was repeatedly raped by a neighbour who lived in a house that later the local children taught her to avoid.

"I knew not to go down that street," she told me. "The other kids would say, 'Don't go down that way,' and I didn't."

Joanna would have been only two years old when her brother was thirteen. Had he told her this story privately, when she was older? Was it another buried family secret that her parents knew too? There's no one now for me to ask.

I WAS AFRAID of forgetting who my mother had been before her illness took root in her. I began to reach out to a few of her old friends, like the guy from her art school days, like her friend from high school. I emailed the editor of *Beowulf to Beatles*, letting him know how much his anthology meant to my mother and me, and I emailed an underground filmmaker who had been one of my mother's professors, the one who had played the John Giorno track in class. Both men wrote back, but their generous responses didn't hold any new clues about my mother's past and I let our correspondences die out.

As I looked people up, I realized that even people my own age were disappearing. My old friend Andrea, whom I'd hoped to call, though I hadn't seen her in years, had sent me a message on Facebook after seeing a post about my mother. *Just wanted to send a little spark of light and a shout out to you—it sounds like your mom isn't doing well. I remember Joanna as being this positive point of light from that time in my life*, she wrote. *I envied the creative energy and joy that was in your house.* We had a brief, warm exchange and when I reached out again a couple of years later, Andrea's Facebook page was filled with memorial tributes. I found an obituary online; she had died months after sending me that message, from "complications of pneumonia." I was stunned. Around the same time, my cousin Ann died of cancer.

I ran into roadblocks when I tried to find some of my mother's exes. I don't know if I ever knew Eddie's last name, for example, the young cook at the pizza parlour whom I loved as a child.

Ironically, my father had become one of the last available sources of information about my mother's history.

Joanna, though, continued to surprise me. One day, when I was visiting with Levi in tow, she asked me for a favour. "Do you know how to get in touch with your father?" she asked me.

"I do," I told her, startled. She hadn't mentioned my father in years.

"He was a good daddy," she said, with a childlike sweetness. "My sister was jealous and she told me to leave him. But I shouldn't have left him. He loved us, he took care of us."

"Oh," I said. Levi was at my feet, throwing the pieces of a puzzle all over the floor. There were three or four boxes of puzzles, featuring various bucolic scenes, stored under the television in the small lounge where we sat. I bent down to gather up some wayward cardboard fragments depicting microscopic sprays of lavender. I had never heard her speak of my father this way.

Joanna's voice turned coy. "I mean, he probably got married . . ." she said, looking at me out of the corner of her eye.

"Well, yes," I told her tentatively, "he is married. He's been married a long time."

"Oh," she said, deflating. "Oh. Well, never mind, then."

The only other evidence I ever had of the depth of my mother's affection for my father was in that letter she had written to him in the late summer of 1971. In it, she did everything she could to convince him to join her in Michigan. She calculated figures again and again, obsessively outlining what she could do with the money she was making, working at a department store. She wrote that she wanted to make him the beneficiary of her life insurance but couldn't do so because they weren't married. Over and over, she referenced money she owed him. She wanted him so badly. In all our years together, I never knew her to want anyone as badly as she wanted my father in this letter. She'd had countless affairs, and a few boyfriends, and once or twice after I'd left home she got a little hung up on someone who treated her poorly, like that last guy she dated in Michigan—but she had bounced back from those disappointments with relative ease. She'd never talked about how great any of them were. She was, I imagine, determined not to lose herself so completely ever again, never to humiliate herself so much over a man.

It was a shock for me to see how far gone she was in this letter.

This was also a shock: she must have known she was pregnant when she wrote the letter, but she didn't tell him.

The night after I read it, I couldn't sleep, haunted by the intensity of my mother's words. I crept out of bed around three in the morning and wrote two poems arranging language I lifted straight from her letter. It was like solving a puzzle, discovering how the lines might fit together in a new, truer order. I was digging out the story underneath the story. As I was writing the second poem, the sun began to rise. The only line of my own is, "Suddenly, it's light outside."

SONGS TO SING TO AN ESTRANGED LOVER WHILE SECRETLY PREGNANT

Darling I Miss You Why Don't You Write Song
I Will Pay You Back Some of What I Owe You for Countless
   Things Song
My Cooking Problem Song
Scorpio Loves Hates Fights and Endures Song
Pisces Responds Instantly to a Call for Help Song
I Feel Like Running Away North and Hiding under a Rock Song
I Wish I Could Write Straight Song
Book on Reincarnation Song
I'm Trying to Be So Good to Persuade You Song
Even the Shrink Says We Shouldn't Get Married Song
Jobs Are Opening Up Song
We Lost but Played a Fantastic Game Song
Priceless Nephew Song
Cup of Strong Coffee Song
Do You Still Wear Your Cross Song
I Want You Please Be Good Song
I'm Going to Pay the $60 Bill Song
Plane Fare Song
Work Today Tomorrow Off Song
Suddenly It's Light Outside Song
Filling Out Forms Song
Learning Rules Song
$70 a Week Song
X-Ray and Wisdom Teeth Song
Life Insurance Song
Eating Constantly Still Weighing 103 Song

Body Cramps during Exercise and Gets Tired Song
Have to Flatten My Stomach Song
Firm My Breasts and Tush Song
I Need a Magician Song
Old Family Farm Song
Land Going for $300 an Acre Song
Corn 13 Inches Long Song
Mashed Potato Song
Homemade Bread Song
Homegrown Apples Song
Ten-Room House Song
In the Family 100 Years Song
Dream of European Travel Song
Come Soon Song
Come Soon Song
If I Wasn't So Healthy I'd Think I Was Dying Song

wager / wagon / waif / waist / waiter / waiver

walker / wall / waltz / wand / wanderer

want / war / ward / wardrobe / warning

warrant / warts / washer / wasp / waste

water / watercolour / wave / wax / way

weakness / wealth / weapon / weather

weaving / web / wedding / wedge / weed

weeks / weeper / weight / welcome / welfare

whale / whatnot / wheel / whip / whirl

whisker / whistle / wickedness / wife / wiggle

wilderness / wildflowers / will / willingness

willow / wind / window / wine / wings / wink

winter / wire / wisdom / wish / witch

withdrawal / W I T N E S S / woe / wolf

woman / wonder / woods / wool / work / world

wormhole / wormwood / worry / worship

worth / wound / wrath / wreath / wreck

wrist / writer / wrongs

MY MOTHER AND I sat on a mauve loveseat in the family room at the end of a long hall on the ground floor of the nursing home. The room was bland, appointed with faded faux-fancy furniture that, despite its wear, still exuded a low shine not on display anywhere else in the building. A large dining room table was surrounded by matching chairs in dark wood; an empty hutch loomed at the far end of the room, the kind used for safekeeping the good dishes. Joanna and I usually sat on the overstuffed loveseat, beside a rolling cart with a stack of Styrofoam cups and an unplugged coffee maker.

Joanna had finally been pushed out of the assisted-living facility where I'd tried to keep her; she had run out the door one day and made it a fair distance down the street before a staff member caught up with her. I could no longer argue the fact that she needed to live in a secure building. The facility refused to move her into one of their nice nursing homes, and it was almost impossible to find a nursing home that would admit her. In addition to not having enough money to buy our way into a decent place, my mother now had a diagnosis of frontal-lobe dementia written in her file. Instead of providing a basis for strategizing her care, that diagnosis only served to blackball my mother at facilities that had been burned before by difficult residents. I was pressured to move Joanna into a rundown nursing home, because, I was told, "If you don't agree to this, she could end up someplace much, much worse." I was assured it might look a little shabby around the edges but the people who worked there were caring. "That's what counts," the administrator of the assisted-living facility told me, as she pushed us out the door. A junior staffer from the assisted-living facility who had grown attached to my mother helped move her few remaining belongings. According to the social worker at my mother's new nursing home, the young woman sobbed through the whole process, but Joanna seemed to take the change in stride.

After years of fighting against this outcome, my greatest fear had come true, and the numbness I felt held a perverse kinship to relief. There was no shoe left to drop.

Whenever I visited my mother during this time, I always brought her to this room, designed to host family gatherings, and it was always empty. On this particular day, Mike had driven me and then he and Levi left, after saying hello to Grandma Jo-Jo. This was the name I gave Levi to call his grandmother. Over the past year we'd all spent hours in this underused visiting room, Levi playing with Lego or small cars or a motorized toy truck. He loved to stack sealed tubs of non-dairy creamer. Joanna would smile as she watched his industriousness. "The baby is so sweet," she'd say, over and over.

The baby was almost four years old now, and he didn't understand why Grandma Jo-Jo called him a baby. Mike and Levi had headed to a nearby park, leaving my mother and me time to sit alone for a couple of hours. I sat close and read aloud to her, choosing poems that I remembered her liking from a copy of the anthology she had owned all those years earlier, *Beowulf to Beatles*, that I'd found on eBay. I read her the lyrics to "Suzanne" by Leonard Cohen and the anonymous ballad "Bar'bra Allen," a melodramatic tale about a man who mysteriously dies after his lover accuses him of slighting her at the village pub. The woman visits his deathbed, carrying her grudge, then goes home and tells her mother, "Oh mother mother make my bed / Make it soft and narrow / Since my love died for me today / I'll die for him tomorrow."

"That's a good one," my mother said when I finished.

And then a shiver passed through her body and she struggled to stand up, a look of panic on her face. It quickly dawned on me what the problem was. "Do you need to go to the bathroom?" I asked her. She nodded. It smelled as if she had already lost control of her bowels. I guided her to the only bathroom I'd ever used in the building, which was inside the staff changing room down the hall. This was a small space with rows of bleak lockers and a couple of toilet stalls behind an interior door. I brought her into one of the stalls and helped her pull down her pants and immediately saw that her pull-up disposable underpants were filled with shit. Her ass was covered in shit.

What language do I have for this experience? The word in my head at the time wasn't *feces*, it was *shit*. Shit, shit, shit, I thought. What do I do?

"It's okay," I told her. "Don't worry about this. I can take care of this. Just wait a second."

Changing my son's diaper instilled me with a sense of competence. Yes, my mother was close to my own height and was now at least forty pounds heavier than me, but still, I reasoned, it was the same thing. The problem was that I didn't have the necessary supplies. I didn't have wipes, I didn't have a clean pair of pull-ups. As gently and carefully as I could, I pulled off my mother's pants and then her soiled disposable—I don't call it a diaper, I can't quite. I made a thick wad of toilet paper and wet it in the sink while she stood naked from the waist down in the stall, calm and obedient. I cleaned her up as best I could and threw the damp, shit-covered toilet paper and her soiled pull-ups in the garbage. After she was as clean as possible, I guided her feet back into her pants and guided the elastic waistband over her hips. I guided her feet back into her shoes, her weight awkwardly resting on my shoulder as I crouched. When we walked out of the stall, I washed my hands with hot water and about six pumps of the pink institutional soap. I led her back into the hall.

In the lobby on the ground floor, I ran into the social worker, a middle-aged white woman with short blond hair, glasses and a pinched look of bottled anger. I spoke to her in a low, calm tone, explaining the situation.

"I'll get someone to clean her up," she said.

"No," I said, "I want to do it. She needs a bath, and I want to be the one to give it to her. I don't want her to feel like she did anything wrong, or that I'm handing her over to someone else to deal with it. I can deal with it. Is that okay, can I give her a bath?"

"Sure, just tell someone on the floor you need a towel," the woman said, her face impassive over her delicate gold necklace with its delicate gold cross.

When we stepped off the elevator onto the fourth floor, no one was sitting at the nurses' station. Finally, I stopped an aide pushing a cart of towels down the hall. "I need a towel for my mother," I explained. He looked confused but handed me a frayed grey towel.

The shower room was just that, a small room with a drain in the middle of the floor and a hand-held shower nozzle attached to the wall. No soap, no linens, no chair where I could put my mother's clothes to keep them dry. I was relieved to see a box of pull-ups at least.

I undressed my mother and pushed my sleeves up. "It's okay, Mom, I can take care of this."

"You're an angel," she said.

The water coming out of the hand-held shower nozzle was too cold. When it hit the skin on my mother's leg, she jolted up as if she had been struck. "Sorry, Mom," I said. "Let me get it warmer." The water pressure was weak, but after several minutes it trickled over my hand at room temperature.

Though my mother's hair was still dark brown, her pubic hair was grey and matted, and everything about her now was round. Her eyes, her face, her stomach, her legs—all round and pale and dimpled as a child's illustration of the moon. There were no washcloths and so I used my hands to rub water over her dimpled thighs, her swollen ankles, wiping and rinsing the skin around her ass as completely as I could. I kept talking as we did this, as if we were still sitting on the loveseat. I joked about the water. "I didn't mean to scare you with that cold water! What was I thinking?" I said, speaking like an actress in a sitcom. I made my voice a little louder, every gesture a little bigger, my smile and laugh cues that it was time for her to do the same.

"You're an angel," she said again.

An angel wouldn't leave you here and go home, I thought. An angel would carry you away from this dump, not incompetently bathe you.

I pulled nail clippers and hand cream out of my purse and clipped her thick, yellowed toenails while she stood, the towel not quite big enough to wrap around her hips like a sarong. I rubbed her feet with the hand cream. I couldn't find a wastebasket, so I left the nail clippings on the floor in a tidy pile. I dried her with the ratty towel and when I reached for her clothes, which I had stashed in a far corner, I realized that I'd managed to get her socks wet. I didn't like the idea of her walking back to her room barefoot, so I struggled to get the shaggy synthetic, and now damp, socks back on her feet.

A little later, as I was waiting alone by the main exit for Mike and Levi to return for me, one of the women who worked in the facility came up to me. "Did you throw out that disposable in our bathroom? That's the staff's bathroom," she said.

"I'm sorry, I didn't know what else to do," I said. But by that time, I was not all that sorry.

❦

AS WE DROVE home, Levi fell asleep in the car seat. Up front with Mike, I watched the lights of the freeway flashing by, one after another. When I shut my eyes, I saw my mother's body standing before me in the shower, soft and cold.

The next morning, Mike came into my office upstairs, carrying a cup of hot coffee. I was sitting at my desk, a stack of my mother's notebooks and sketchbooks beside me. They were filled with drawings of babies, drawings of rabbits, drawings of rabbits acting like babies.

"Here, come look at this drawing my mother made," I said to him, holding up a soft ink-wash image of a faceless female figure wearing a form-fitting dress and holding what I assumed was a small, dark purse, an evening bag, against her hip. There was another figure as well, almost formless, an echo, but still recognizably feminine in its posture, holding one hand over its right breast and resting the other hand low on its belly.

"I don't know why I find this one so haunting," I said to Mike, turning around in my chair. The coffee steamed in my hand as I watched him gaze at the drawing. A few seconds passed.

"Disappearing woman, dude," he said.

What didn't I see
What didn't I see
What didn't I see

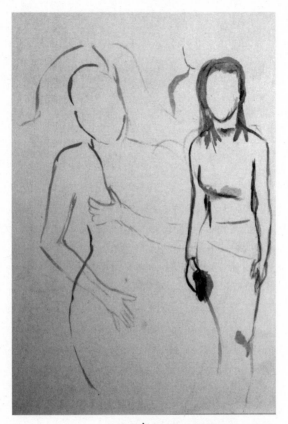

JOANNA'S SKETCHBOOK, UNDATED

yack / yammer / yard / yarn / yearbook
yearning / years / yeast / yell / yellowjacket
yes-man / yesterday / yield / yoga / yoke
yolk / Y O U T H

IN THE FALL of 2018, I spent six weeks renting an empty apartment from a friend, trying to make a narrative out of the fragments of my mother's life, her remaining treasures spread about me: pictures propped against the walls, books piled up on the floor, decoupaged blocks stacked along the back of the writing desk.

"You know, your mom's stuff—" my friend said when she came into the room, looking around slowly. "These are the possessions of a child."

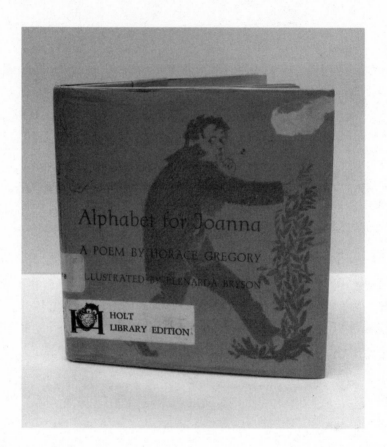

Alphabet for Joanna

A POEM BY HORACE GREGORY

ILLUSTRATED BY LEONARD A. BRYSON

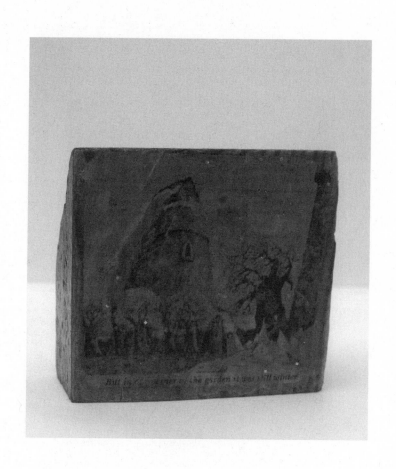

But in the corner of the garden it was still winter.

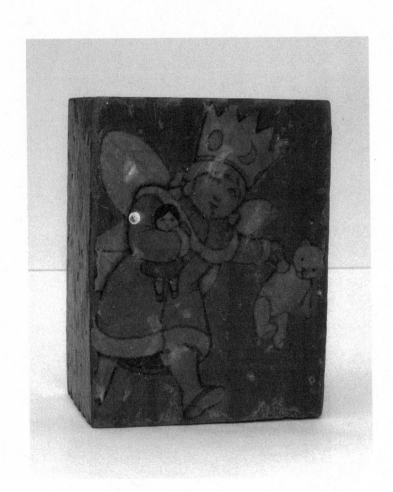

Missing: Melvin, a sienna-coloured teddy bear with loose-button eyes and loved-down fur. He belonged first to Joanna's older sister, and then to Joanna. The siblings had squabbled for decades over the question of whose house the bear belonged in. Joanna did not begrudge her sister's claim, though she missed Melvin as if he were a lost brother.

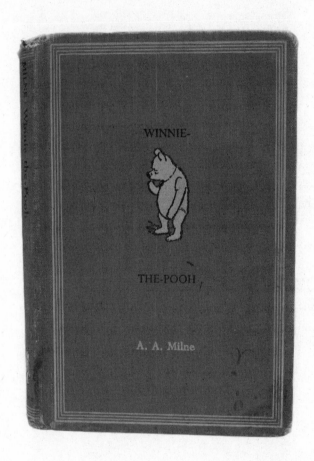

WINNIE-

THE-POOH

A. A. Milne

WINNIE-

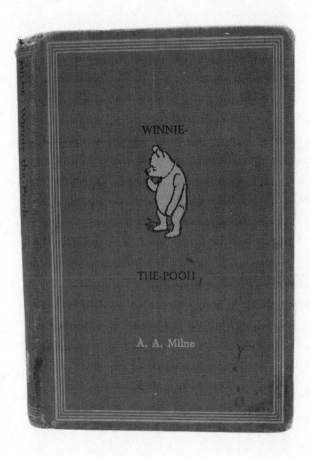

THE-POOH

A. A. Milne

Missing: Melvin, a sienna-coloured teddy bear with loose-button eyes and loved-down fur. He belonged first to Joanna's older sister, and then to Joanna. The siblings had squabbled for decades over the question of whose house the bear belonged in. Joanna did not begrudge her sister's claim, though she missed Melvin as if he were a lost brother.

donnie, it's a very strange thing to give you, I have the other half of the set, but I want you to have it because I'm half of a set because I love you, because you're you.

love, jo

fable / face / facility / factions / faculties / failure
fairies / fairness / faith / fall / family / fantasy
farm / fatality / fate / F A T H E R / fault
fear / fence / ferocity / ferry / fever / fiction
fidelity / fight / files / finality / fingers / fire / fish
fitness / flame / flashback / flasher / flight / flirt
flood / floor / flour / flower / focus / fog / folders
font / force / forcefield / forest / forgetfulness
formation / forms / fort / fortune / foundling
fox / foxglove / fracture / fragment / framework
fray / freak / freedom / frenzy / friends / fright
frost / fruit / fugitive / fullness / fumble / fun
function / fuse / future

Scene: A woman in her forties sits inside a screened-in porch at a small wooden table. She is writing in a notebook. Through the black wire screens, we can see that the porch is surrounded by a tight circle of tall trees. Though it's nearly noon, the room is lit in a dappled green light.

We hear the sound of a car pulling up the long rocky driveway, wheels crunching closer.

The woman walks offstage, then returns alongside a man carrying a large cardboard box in both arms.

FATHER: Wow, when you said it was in the woods, you weren't kidding.

The man's hair is grey, and there are pale scars scratched across his cheeks. He is dressed in a pair of clean jeans. A gold chain glints beneath the neckline of his T-shirt. The words on his T-shirt read: I'M CDO:

IT'S LIKE OBSESSIVE-COMPULSIVE DISORDER EXCEPT WITH THE LETTERS IN THE RIGHT ORDER. He sets the box down on the table, on top of the notebook. The woman slides the notebook out from under the box and keeps it in her hands.

Inside the box: a handsome, handmade chessboard; a two-inch-square black plastic tile with a white peace sign burned into it; worn cloth-bound volumes of War and Peace *and* Anna Karenina; *a couple of handfuls of individually wrapped green tea bags; two bars of Irish Spring soap.*

F A T H E R : I woke at four-something in the morning—it was a bathroom call—and decided I wasn't going to fall back asleep.

The man watches as the woman sifts through the contents of the box with one hand, while holding her notebook in the other.

F A T H E R : Your grandfather made that chessboard. I figured Levi should have it. Your mother had painted pieces onto wooden dowels that your grandfather made. I think I have a couple of them still, somewhere . . .

The man pulls out the black plastic tile and hands it to the woman, who turns it over in her hand. She sees it has an adhesive backing, protected by a square sheet of wax paper.

F A T H E R : Your mother had a friend who was burning these peace signs into decals. I thought you might like it.

The man points to the Tolstoy novels in the box.

FATHER: I bought these books with your grandmother at a used bookstore in Royal Oak. We each bought one and she tried to talk me into letting her buy both, and then, somehow [*laughing*], I managed to leave their house with both of them.

The man picks up a book that is lying on the seat of an armchair.

FATHER: Oh, *The Little Prince.*

DAUGHTER: Have you read it?

FATHER: Well, your mother introduced me to it . . .

The woman and the man continue into the house and settle themselves at a large wooden table off the kitchen. They both appear nervous. The woman is still holding her notebook, which she writes in as they talk.

DAUGHTER: I was hoping you could tell me what you remember about my mother from when you were together.

FATHER: Well, she was my Avon lady, that's how we met. We struck up a friendship, drank tea. It was a gradual process over a period of weeks. She was emaciated when I met her, probably eighty-five pounds. She wasn't eating. I'm hesitant—she's your mother. I've been protective. I didn't know what you knew.

DAUGHTER: It's okay, I know a fair bit already.

FATHER: From what your mother told me, her husband was putting aluminum foil on the windows, he was engaging in this hyper-suspicious activity. She alluded to him pushing her . . . She didn't feel safe around him. She moved in with me pretty quick. Your mother and her husband had been married by the reverend of enlightened something or other. I'm not sure how legitimate the actual marriage was.

DAUGHTER: Well, it was legitimate enough that they did have to get divorced. But I don't think it was a complicated process. She told me the fact that I wasn't his child was included in the divorce papers, even though she'd left his name on my birth certificate. What was your relationship like when you lived together in California?

FATHER: Okay, so, after a while, we were fighting, and she and I went to a couples counselling type of thing. Your mom decided, I don't need this crap. The counsellor was really concerned, he took me aside. He could see there was something not quite right, there was something going on. "You need to keep coming back," he told me. "You don't know everything that is going on here." But we didn't go back and things between us were starting to unravel.

DAUGHTER: And then my mother went back to Michigan.

FATHER: Your mom went back to Michigan. After I found out she was pregnant, your grandfather said to me on the phone, "Marry her or don't bother coming out here." He was looking for me to make some kind of commitment. For which I don't blame him. So I went out there and gave it an honest shot, but she would withdraw into this fantasy life. She needed the structure of your grandparents' house to take care of you. Sometimes she couldn't even make it to the store, the laundromat . . . She would become withdrawn, absent. Childlike. She only wanted to do the fun things. I think she was depressed. And we didn't have any money. Everything went into the diapers and the rent.

DAUGHTER: So we all lived with my grandparents for six months, and then the three of us lived in our own apartment for six months after that. And you broke up in January, a year after I was born.

FATHER: I was a Southern California kid in Michigan, freezing my ass off. I was ill-equipped. I didn't have the right clothes. What kicked everything over is when I got fired from my job. That job was pretty dangerous. A big tool-and-die shop in Warren. We were working under dangerous circumstances, working on big jobs from the Big Four. Rooftop panels for the pickup trucks, firewalls. Our parts went to the big assembly plants. But we were using old equipment. We got the old machines when other factories were being upgraded. Some of these machines, when they moved a big load, the whole floor would shake. There were big rubber-belt-run machines that were supposed to have guards on them but didn't. What happened was that the safety department came through and slapped a $10,000 fine on the factory to clean up its act. There was a group of us wanting to form a union. I signed cards of intent with about thirty other guys. We all lost our jobs. That's when your mother left me and our apartment in Detroit for good. That same week.

DAUGHTER: How much do you know about what happened with Allan?

FATHER: When we were living at your grandparents', your grandfather implied she'd already been through enough trauma. I told him I knew about the incident with her brother. I think that brought him up short a bit. He said, "Well, she must really trust you if she shared that." Even your grandmother alluded to it, in a way. I remember one time she said, "Don't ever get in the way of a mother and her child, because it will create a schism." The episode with Joanna's brother really affected her parents' marriage. Your grandfather wanted to kill the guy, and your grandmother wanted to protect him. Your grandmother's attitude was: he may be damaged, but he's my damaged son. She kicked your grandpa out of the bedroom and that was it.

DAUGHTER: I didn't know when they moved into separate rooms. I assumed it was after the kids had all moved out.

FATHER: The rape was seismic in its impact on everyone. Your mom was ground zero. Nothing was the same after that. There was the taboo, there was the act itself. The fallout, the uproar, the reverberations. I get the impression your mother was bruised up. It must have been horrific. To be honest with you, I'm reluctant to say anything mean, but I kind of feel as if your mother might have shared that with me to lock me in—like, now I'm obliged to stay with her. Obligated. Like, "I've shared my darkest secret," or whatever. I don't know, it's hard to interpret someone else's motives. I found what she told me shocking. I didn't share it with anyone. Your relationship with your mother is a sacred thing. I wouldn't want to affect your opinion of her. I met your uncle, and you know it seemed to me that he suffered from bouts of depression.

DAUGHTER: I remember not liking the way he looked at me when I was little, but I didn't have language for it. I couldn't stand being around him.

FATHER: You were striking . . . you still are. You look a lot like your mother.

DAUGHTER: What else do you remember about what she said about the rape?

FATHER: When your mother told me what had happened, I was uncomfortable and she was a little tearful. She was afraid that it might diminish my opinion of her. I could tell it was painful for her. I didn't . . . I didn't ask her to tell me the gory details. We never really talked about it again. Why did she tell me? I don't know. I don't know if it was just to bond with me, to share, to exhibit the degree to which she cared, or . . . to show her investment in her relationship with me. I don't think that there were very many people she would have trusted that to . . .

DAUGHTER: You'd mentioned on the phone that she spent the nights when you were working drinking coffee and smoking cigarettes and drawing. Do you remember what her artwork looked like?

FATHER: I remember she did some drawings inspired by Tolkien; we were both reading the *Lord of the Rings* trilogy. In her fragments of verse and her drawings, there was a dreamlike quality. I guess maybe a fantasy engagement. Adolescent, romantic. I'm not sure. Where does imagination leave off and delusion pick up?

DAUGHTER: Well—

The woman begins to kick her right foot back and forth under her chair.

FATHER: I loved her, and then I fell out of love with her. This is my excuse, alibi, rationale. All I can tell you is that things were bad in Detroit, when your mother went back to your grandparents'. I can tell you that it wouldn't have worked. You had a much better situation with your grandparents than you would have had with your mother and me trying and trying to make a go of it.

DAUGHTER: Oh, please don't misunderstand. I don't think there's any way you and my mother could have stayed together.

FATHER: Okay.

DAUGHTER: My problem—what I think that my mother could never forgive—was that you were able to just walk away from me. I know our lives are completely different, but if Mike and I had split up when Levi was a baby, there's no way he could've walked away from his son.

FATHER: I came to see you a couple times and I got a pretty cold reception from your grandmother. She didn't think much of me after things didn't work out with your mother, which was fair enough, I guess. I probably should have worked harder to maintain a relationship with you. And that's my fault.

The man and the woman are silent for a moment.

FATHER: Was I in love with your mom? I don't know. I cared for her. She had a highly flirtatious nature. She had a sensual way of walking down the street. My friends thought she was flirting with them—it made them uncomfortable. She craved attention. She was very seductive, very alluring. She was witty, learned. We had long, in-depth conversations. When it ended, I was glad to be out from under the responsibility of your mom, but heartbroken at losing you. You were about the only bright spot in my otherwise dreary existence. My mother maintained a connection with your mother. Which made me think that my own mom had a child no one knew about. I'm the only son. I'm not necessarily the best son, but I was the only son. She basically made me feel that I was honour-bound to see what I could do. A lot of mothers would say just forget it, don't jeopardize—

The woman puts down her notebook.

DAUGHTER: I don't know that a lot of mothers would say just forget it.

FATHER: You don't think so? Most mothers are protective. I think most mothers would say, that's *her* problem. I don't know.

DAUGHTER: Maybe your mother did have a child that she'd had to give up, I don't know. But I don't think it's so unusual for people to feel a connection to their son's children, even when the circumstances aren't ideal. I guess I find it difficult to understand how you were able to walk away from me. Knowing we all lived together for a year actually makes it more difficult for me to understand.

The man looks at the table.

FATHER: I don't know that I understand it myself. I feel bad for you. I feel bad for me! I'm not a bad person. There were all these forces. The last time I came to see you, your grandmother went into her room and slammed the door. And I only had a couple bucks and your mom was mad I didn't give her more money. And it was like, okay, yeah, you're right, I probably need to provide. But I was overwhelmed.

DAUGHTER: My mother said I had started talking and then, after you left, I stopped. And that when I started again, it was with new words. Do you remember what my first word was?

FATHER: I don't know. *Dada?*

The woman writes this down. The stage goes dark.

Later, offstage, the FATHER sends the DAUGHTER an email. His feelings are hurt. He has been thinking about some of the things she said and he is disturbed. The daughter had suggested that her mother had not been his biggest fan. The daughter had speculated that maybe her mother had visited her ex while the father was at work. He is wondering. He has to ask.

   Are you sure I am your father?

ulcer / ultimatum / umbrage / umbrella
uncertainty / uncle / unconsciousness
underground / understanding / undertone
undertow / unicorn / U N I O N / unit
universe / university / upheaval / upstairs
urchin / urgency / urine / urn / use / usher
uterus / utility / utopia / utterance

IT TOOK A year and a half, but after filling out dozens of applications, after meeting and sweet-talking countless admissions coordinators, I finally hired a small counselling firm to help me, and after a few months and about a thousand dollars, my mother was accepted into a decent nursing home in a suburb close to the border. I had knocked and knocked and knocked and I'd heard no and no and no, and then one day, as if a switch had been flipped, the answer was yes. Your mother can move in tomorrow.

The new nursing home, with its sunny front atrium, its enclosed courtyard garden and its part-time music therapist, after a year and a half in a place that had been profiled in a local news exposé on their rat infestation, felt in comparison like the solid-gold mansion a kid dreams they would buy if they won the lottery. Even Joanna, who could barely communicate through language at this point, was visibly grateful when I told her, yes, this was her new home.

I'll never know if the stress of the previous institution contributed to an acceleration of her decline, but by the time she settled into the new nursing home, my mother could no longer carry on even a simple conversation. On one particular day when I arrived for a visit, I found Joanna sitting in the lounge, in a chair by the window, holding her black slip-on sneakers in her lap. Like most of the other residents, she was wearing socks issued by the facility. They were a kind of pale green-blue, that colour that was once the unflattering shade of choice for bridesmaid dresses—what my mother would call seafoam. They had a synthetic plush texture, a shaggy pile like the fur of a cheap stuffed animal, and somehow the soles were always dirty—perhaps because many of the residents walked around the locked unit in sock feet.

Joanna put one of her black slip-on sneakers on the side table beside her. There was a handle on the front of this table to suggest a drawer where small treasures might be stored, and my mother pulled on the handle. But it was only decorative; there was no drawer at all. Joanna looked down at the other shoe in her lap, lifted it to her face and sniffed it.

I carefully collected both slip-ons and placed them on the floor before her feet, smiling at her. "Do you want to wear your shoes?" I asked.

She looked at me and then slid her feet into them. Almost immediately, she took them off again.

An aide came by to ask if my mother would like to have her food on a tray in the lounge, as they were serving dinner. "I thought maybe you two would like to sit together here, instead of going into the dining room," the woman said to me.

Joanna didn't respond, but I agreed that it would be nicer for us to stay where we were. The aide set down a tray with plates under plastic covers, which I removed. I watched as my mother tasted a gelatinous orange-brown pudding (butterscotch, I guessed) and then spread it thickly onto her tuna fish sandwich. I watched as she deconstructed her sandwich, pulling the bread away and rolling the gummy white sheets into balls, eating some, discarding others. I watched as she tentatively stabbed with her fork the plush paw of a robotic pet cat that I'd placed on the table. I watched as she ate some of the "broccoli salad"—thankfully, recognizably a vegetable, though it was coated in a gluey white sauce.

When Joanna was first diagnosed, it was easier to think about her death than it was to imagine how all of us might live with this. Back then, I had googled the average life expectancy of a person suffering frontal-lobe dementia. Seven years. How will we make it, I'd thought at the time.

Just shoot me. Her words echoing in my ears.

❧

I TOLD MYSELF that I wished for my mother to die out of a sense of mercy. But I also didn't know how I could stand it, watching her slowly vanish bit by bit, year by year.

Even so, for a long time I didn't want to sign a do-not-resuscitate order. Every quarter, medical staff would call and ask if I wanted to sign one. One year they called me the day after Christmas. "Do you still want us to revive your mother if . . ."

Finally, when Joanna landed in the hospital after a seizure, a doctor walked me through the process. Mike stood close beside me as this doctor asked me about my mother's directives. Had I thought about changing the standing order to a DNR?

For the first time someone took me aside to speak to me about what these directives meant. This doctor's bedside manner was the best I'd ever encountered. He was probably around my age, maybe even younger; he wore his authority loosely, comfortably, and I accepted it without question. He explained why inserting a feeding tube, in the event that Joanna couldn't swallow on her own, would be a pointless cruelty. "She wouldn't have the pleasure of eating, of tasting her food," he said.

I thought of my mother smearing butterscotch pudding on her tuna fish sandwich.

"I'm not sure how much pleasure she's getting out of eating now . . . but if she didn't have the tube, would she starve?" I asked.

The doctor gently turned page after page, explaining terms, pointing: here, sign here, and here. As I made a careful *X* inside each of the small boxes at which he pointed, tears slid down my cheeks, but I did not make a sound.

❦

YEARS AGO, AFTER I had graduated from university, I hung around the college town of Ann Arbor, cleaning houses here and there for the little bit of money I needed to get by in the summer. I found my clients—although I would never have used the word *clients* then—from the university job board.

Mrs. Fredericks, one of those clients, suffered from a degenerative disease. She had lost the ability to speak, so we communicated through a three-party call. She typed out what she wanted to say, and a woman receiving the transmissions would read her words back to me.

She was a thin white woman, very erect, and wore a scarf wrapped around her head, turban-style. Her house was small and well-maintained, neat and full of light. She wrote out how she wanted the house cleaned on a yellow pad of paper.

I was nervous and awkward around her, and she didn't like that. I talk more loudly when I'm anxious. "I'm not deaf," she wrote on the yellow pad.

One day her daughter came by while I was cleaning and I watched them together. I thought I picked up on some kind of static between them, though the daughter was friendly with me.

Mrs. Fredericks never called me to clean again after that. I've always felt a little ashamed about it. I'd failed a test.

Months later, while staying with Joanna for a couple of months before moving to London, I saw a photograph of Mrs. Fredericks on the evening news. She had inhaled carbon monoxide through a mask attached to a "suicide machine" designed and operated by Dr. Kevorkian. I was stunned.

When Joanna came home from work, I told her what I had seen on the news. I remember sitting on the blue-and-green floral couch, petting Tasha, the fluffy black cat my mother had bought me for Christmas the year before I'd left for school. It was her cat now. Joanna disappeared down the hall for a few minutes. When she returned, she said, "Listen, I want to tell you something. I signed a living will. If I ever end up in a car accident or something like that, I want you to pull the plug. I don't want to be a vegetable." She gave me a hard look. "You'll be the one who has to make the decision. Do you understand?"

Yes, I told her. I understood.

❦

AFTER JOANNA HAD been discharged from the hospital, after I had signed all the papers for the DNR directive, I met with the care manager of the nursing home about what would happen when my mother died.

"Honestly, I pray that my residents have a heart attack," the care manager said. She was in her late twenties or early thirties, fresh-faced and casually dressed. Her nail polish was chipped, just like mine.

"What happened to that guy my mother used to sit next to? Lenny?" I asked. Lenny was tall and his hair was always slicked back in a subtle pompadour. Mike had fondly called him "the greaser."

"Oh, he passed," the care manager told me. This surprised me, as Lenny hadn't looked old, though he had been in a wheelchair the last time I'd seen him. "I used to put your mother next to him when he was agitated," she continued, "and he would calm right down. It was great."

After our meeting, I found Joanna in the lounge, and I led her back to her room so that we could listen to music. Music was still the most effective way for me to connect to her. Even though she no longer spoke in clear sentences, she could hum and sing along to familiar songs. Musical memories are linked to areas of the brain that are often less affected by dementia, so that patients who no longer speak are sometimes able to sing. I chased these moments of connection, though I never knew how long they would hold—the flash of fragile clarity was so intense, and it always passed away as suddenly as it arrived.

I remembered how we used to sing "Across the Universe," from our *Beatles Songbook*, back when Joanna had first bought her guitar. I pulled up a remastered version on Spotify and pressed play. Immediately, Joanna began to sway in time to the song, mumbling the first lines.

"Nothing's gonna change my world," we sang when we reached the chorus, and as we locked eyes, there she was. Joanna. She knew me. She knew the words. She knew what the words meant. Her eyes welled up with tears and she drew a jagged breath, but she didn't break eye contact as we leaned into each other, our heads bowed, foreheads touching, my arms gripping her arms. Together we insisted, again and again, "Nothing's gonna change my world—"

"Mom, I'm so sorry," I said, and we both wept.

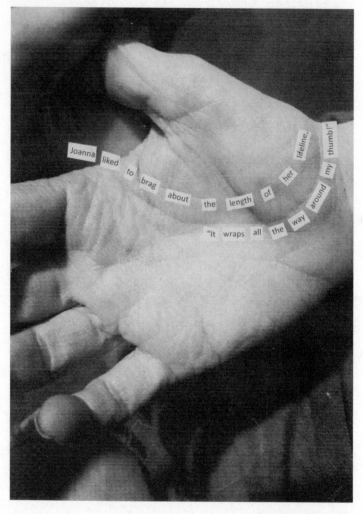

Joanna liked to brag about the length of her lifeline, "It wraps all the way around my thumb!"

JOANNA'S HAND, 2017

cabaret / cabinet / cable / caboodle / cachet
cacophony / cadence / caduceus / caesura / cage
cake / cakewalk / calamity / calculations / caldron
calendar / call / calligraphy / callous / calm / cameo
camera / camisole / camomile / campground
campus / canal / cancellation / candidate / candle
candour / candy / cantaloupe / canvas / capacity
cape / capital / caprice / capsules / captive / car
carbon / card / cardinal / career / caregiver
carnation / carnival / carrier / cartomancy
cartoons / case / cash / castaway / castle / cataclysm
catalogue / catastrophe / catcall / categorization
cats / cause / caution / cave / caveat / ceiling
celerity / celibacy / cell / cemetery / centaur / centre
cents / century / ceramics / cerebellum / cerebrum
ceremony / certification / cervix / chain / chair
challenge / chamber / chameleon / champion
change / channels / chant / chaperone / charisma
charts / chasm / chastity / chats / cheapness / cheater
check / chemical / cheque / chess / chest / chevalier
chiffon / child / childbirth / childhood / chimeras
chocolate / choice / choir / chord / chore / chorus
C H R O N O L O G Y / church / cigarettes
cinders / cipher / circle / circumstance / citadel
citizen / city / civilian / civility / clairvoyant
clash / clasp / class / claw / clay / cleaners / clincher
clinic / cloisters / close-ups / cloud / clover / clues
clumsiness / coast / code / coercion / coffee
cognition / cohesion / coins / coldness / collaboration
collage / collapse / collection / collusion / colour

column / combination / comforter / comfrey
commitment / commotion / communication
community / compact / companion / comparison /
compartment / compassion / compatibility /
compensation / competence / competition /
complaint / complex / complication / compliments /
composition / composure / compromise / compulsion
/ computer / concealment / concentration /
conception / concession / conclusion / condemnation
/ condescension / conditions / confession / confidant
/ confidence / confinement / confiscation / conflict /
conformity / confrontation / confusion / conjurer /
connections / conscience / consciousness /
conscription / consent / conspirator / constancy /
constellation / constraint / constriction /
consultation / contact / content / contract /
contribution / control / conure / convalescent /
convert / cookbook / copy / cord / corduroy / corner /
corona / corporation / correction / corridor / cortex
/ cortisol / cosmetics / cosmos / costs / costume /
counsel / cousin / covetousness / co-workers / crack /
cradle / cranium / crash / craving / crayons / crease
/ creation / credit / creep / crepe / crest / crevice /
crib / crisis / criteria / critic / crone / cross / crow /
crowd / cruise / crumbs / crusade / crust / cry /
crystal / cub / cubicle / cuddle / culpability / cult /
cultivation / culture / cunning / cup / cure / curfew
/ curio / curiosity / currents / curse / curveball /
cushion / custody / cutbacks / cycle / cymbal / cyst

Joanna Katherine is born in Billings, Montana, Yellow- 1949
stone County, October 29. Scorpio. On her birth certificate: "Father: 33, white, salesman at Laurel Trading
Co. Mother: 33, white." What make of car kicks up
dust on the drive home to their little house? What
colour sky? She arrives home from the hospital on
Halloween, in time for the family to hand out candy to
the kids who come to the door.

After the family leaves Montana, Joanna and her siblings 1951
stay with their paternal grandmother in Pennsylvania for
the summer, while their father looks for a job and house
in Michigan. The town where Joanna's grandmother lives
is so small that there are no numbers on the houses. It is
in this small town, during these months, where, according
to my mother—many years later, after her diagnosis with
dementia—her brother Allan is repeatedly raped by a
neighbour, a man who lives in a house that the local kids
later warn her to avoid. In 1951, Allan is thirteen years old.

On the sidewalk in front of the family's new house in 1952
the Detroit suburbs, Joanna smiles beside her serious
sister, the seeded plot behind them protected by ropes.

Later, Joanna will tell me that she is three years old
when Allan begins to molest her.

Joanna, her parents, her sister and her two brothers cross 1953
the country, car-camping on their first visit to Montana
since moving away. In home movies of this trip, Allan
climbs and sits alone at the peak of a mountainous out-
crop of rock.

Joanna watches as Allan revives an unconscious sparrow 1954
by holding it under a thin stream of water at the sink.
When she sees it start to stir in his hands, she believes
he has brought the bird back to life.

1955	Lying on her stomach in the living room, Joanna sings along to the theme song of *The Mickey Mouse Club*. How often is she alone with Allan?

1955   Lying on her stomach in the living room, Joanna sings along to the theme song of *The Mickey Mouse Club*. How often is she alone with Allan?

1956   Allan joins the navy at the age of seventeen, and he and Joanna never live in the same house again. Joanna will soon turn seven years old.

1957   While watching the children's television show *Captain Kangaroo*, Joanna falls in love with Lamb Chop, a sock puppet with the face of a sheep and the personality of a sassy but vulnerable six-year-old girl.

1958   On a second family trip back to her grandparents' ranch in Montana, this time without Allan, Joanna befriends a palomino mare that won't let anyone else near her or her colt.

1963   Joanna and her two best friends at school bond over their determination to one day move to London, England, where they will each marry a Beatle—or at least find a cool scene. They walk the halls at school like they know something no one else understands.

1964   Joanna watches a roselike cluster of pink balloons float above her as she screams alongside thousands of other teenaged girls, their voices obliterating the sound of the Beatles singing "You Can't Do That." Some months later, Joanna is raped by her brother Allan. She runs to her friend's house, who will later remember Joanna as being distraught, her clothes "dishevelled." The *Americans 1963* travelling exhibition of fifteen painters and sculptors, including the work of Marisol Escobar alongside Claes Oldenburg, James Rosenquist and other famous male artists, opens at the Detroit Institute of Arts. After seeing it, Joanna dreams of one day being a woman and an artist like Marisol.

On August 13, Joanna returns to Olympia Stadium to see the Beatles live. She still can't hear a note over the screams of fans.

1966

On April 30, months before her high school graduation, Joanna attends the Belle Isle Love-In with her boyfriend, the one she will follow to California two years later. In a photo taken at the Love-In, he wears wraparound sunglasses reminiscent of the Velvet Underground. Joanna wears rust corduroy bell-bottoms, and nearly disappears into the side of his body, her eyes wide, dark, nervous as a deer's. Somewhere in the crowd is John Sinclair, manager of the MC5 and founder of the White Panther Party, a circular patch of LSD stuck onto his third eye. Members of the biker gang the Outlaws drink beer and scowl. On a scuffed VW bus someone has painted the word *LOVE*. A guy starting to grow out his hair blows up a balloon stamped with the word *LOVE*. A girl passes out small white cards that read only: *LOVE*. Two months later, the Insurrection Act of 1807 is invoked to justify deploying more than ten-thousand federal troops to Detroit in response to an uprising against the city's long history of anti-Black racism. The Beatles release the song "All You Need Is Love" as a non-album single, and Joanna thinks it's a joke. In her high school senior yearbook, after her name, it lists: Pep Club 2; Art Club 3; Drama Club 4.

1967

Joanna's boyfriend tries to take her to an MC5 show at the Grande Ballroom and the guy at the door won't let them in. "She is WAY too young, man," he says to Joanna's boyfriend, ignoring their protests that she is over eighteen.

1968

Joanna joins her boyfriend in California, where they marry.

1969

Joanna sits on a porch in Long Beach, wearing tight flared blue jeans and an oversized black T-shirt. She's smiling, a little shyly. Barefoot. One hand on her knee,

1970

the other held in the air in a gesture that is hard to read: she is beckoning the photographer, and she is protecting herself from him. Soon she will meet my father.

1971   Back with her parents in Michigan, Joanna writes to my father, noting that she is receiving psychiatric counselling: *I go once a week to get my head shrunk, which means I'm half as crazy as people who go twice a week.* She is pregnant, something she hides from everyone as long as possible. In a photo taken toward the end of the year, Joanna sits in her parents' dining room. Her stomach is obscured by the table. She looks perhaps fourteen, and happy.

1972   Joanna becomes a mother when I am born in January.

1973   Just before or just after my first birthday, Joanna leaves the apartment we lived in with my father and moves back in with her parents. That summer, we see my father for the last time for more than a decade.

1974   Joanna and I continue to live with her parents. She may or may not have begun to work at a pizza joint on Coolidge. I remember red glass lampshades, the rare treat of restaurant food.

1975   In the fall, Joanna enrolls in a ninety-minute evening Life Drawing class at the Center for Creative Studies. She receives a B-minus. She models for a student photographer in a series of photos, appearing topless in a few (which she did not keep). She regrets doing this, because of the way the male students treat her afterward. She keeps one eleven-by-fourteen-inch print of a close-up of her face, distorted by shadows.

1976   Joanna quits smoking and learns how to drive. She dates a man named Eddie, whom I adore. I pet the thick ginger hair on his arms and ask, "When will my fur grow in?"

Eddie cooks pizzas at the restaurant where Joanna wait-
resses. He is eighteen to her twenty-six. I love him. I love
him and I won't remember his last name.

Joanna and I make a papier mâché marionette of a dog   1977
with floppy ears in a ballet costume. We name him
Rudolf Nureyev Dog. She continues to waitress and go
to art school part-time.

Joanna continues to include me in her Saturday drawing   1978
and painting classes. She will later tell me, after she has
been in an assisted-living facility for two years, that she
brought me with her to give my grandmother a break
and also because one of her professors was hitting on her
and she didn't know how to handle it. "He'd come up to
me and I'd say, 'Oh, I can't, I have my daughter here ...'"

Joanna begins to work as a "keyliner" at a publishing   1979
company specializing in trade journals aimed at contrac-
tors. She cuts text into strips with her X-acto knife and
lays them down like thin paper bricks, arranging them
carefully into columns before she hands the page over to
the camera department. She will work here for seventeen years, eventually teaching herself computer graphics programs as they are introduced.

Joanna rents a small house across the street from her par-   1980
ents and we each have our own room. It is the first time
she has ever had a place of her own, a lease in her name;
the first time she's had her own bedroom with a door
since she left home at nineteen. She is now thirty-one.

Joanna tells a supervisor at work that she is not there for   1981
him to paw. He lifts his hands in the air and walks backwards, blinking. She dates a guy who owns a record store.
President Reagan takes office: my grandparents voted for
him; Joanna did not. Joanna helps me make a one-page

newspaper, and buys a half-moon conure as a pet for me; I name him Precious Greenwing. He learns to mimic kissing noises and the human coo of *awwwwww*. He bites all male visitors foolish enough to stick their fingers anywhere within range of his sharp, curved beak. Joanna takes me to church when I decide I want to convert to Catholicism, but she does not convert herself.

1982   Joanna enrolls in advertising classes at Wayne State. She buys coffee-table books: one on the art of the film *The Dark Crystal*, one on fairies, one on gnomes. We move into a larger apartment, a couple of miles away from my grandparents. My mother tells me who my father is. She begins to go on more dates.

1983   *I am sorry for not writing sooner,* Joanna writes my father in a letter postmarked September 19—the earliest-dated letter from her, about me, that I own—*but I am very busy & very bad at letters. Thank you for the money. We have decided to buy her a new coat with it. Her old one fits but looks really worn.* She explains that I am *growing like a weed: she can wear most of my clothes & her feet are bigger* and that *this was the first year we had a real vacation together.* She shares with him the story of how we drove together down to Kansas and Texas to see one of her brothers (not Allan) and her sister. *We camped all the way down. It was very exciting and we felt very brave.* At the end of the letter she adds, *I told her about us—like you suggested last spring, and she took it well. Thanks again for the money.* And then: her signature a flourish of swirls, an unrecognizable *J*.

1984   *Sorry for not writing for so long,* Joanna begins another letter to my father, this one written on December 14. *I've been very busy. I got damian a pr. of jeans and a scarf with the money. Thank you.* She also notes that she has joined the Women's Advertising Club and might take the next semester off school. *We're going to take some dance lessons after Xmas. I got a coupon book that has free dance lessons.* On December 27 she writes again, thanking him for money that she says will *pay for the other half of her swimming.* Before signing off, she adds, *If you would like to come see her, we could arrange something.*

Joanna sees my father for the first time since 1973 when we meet him at a YMCA swim meet in Kalamazoo. I won't see him again for four more years. In the fall, we move to an apartment behind Sunshine Foods, so that I can attend the same high school she did. In a letter to my father, Joanna explains how she is charting family trees from the information her mother had compiled. She's been playing more guitar and might teach me. (I remember Joanna playing guitar with a handsome Polish man who lived in an apartment across the court-yard and had a wife and kid back in the old country.) *I keep telling my mother that I wasn't cut out to be the mother of a teenager & she tells me no one is,* Joanna writes. *We do have our ups & downs. But all in all she's a pretty good kid.*

1985

Joanna buys her first house, with the help of her parents. I begin working summers with my mother, helping with data entry in the circulation department of her office.

1986

Joanna attends her twenty-year high school reunion, proud of how well she has aged in comparison with more popular classmates. She comes back with a boy-friend. She and I share work clothes.

1987

Joanna often spends the night at her boyfriend's house in West Bloomfield—until she reads my diary and grounds me for drinking. This same boyfriend buys me a phone in the shape of a pink high-heeled shoe, crow-ing over how perfect it is for me. I hate it. Joanna sur-prises me with a fluffy black kitten. She chooses a black

1988

cat at the shelter out of concern for them, because she has heard stories about sadists who adopt black cats just to torture them.

1989

After I graduate and leave for university in the fall, Joanna realizes that she doesn't like her boyfriend of two years after all, and breaks off the relationship. In the fall, at Michigan State, I see my father for the first time since the swim meet. My mother and I continue to share work clothes.

1990

Joanna visits me at university every two weeks and takes me to lunch. She buys me a small plastic goldfish at a novelty shop we like. Back at home, she joins a French Club and travels with the group to Montreal for a weekend.

1991

Joanna watches her mother die of cancer in the hospital. At her side are her two brothers, her father and me. (Joanna's sister is visiting Paris, and unable to get back in time.) It is not a peaceful death: my grandmother cries for her mother, her eyes shiny with terror. For the funeral, Joanna asks me to read her favourite passage from *The Little Prince*, because she knows she couldn't read it herself without weeping. In a letter to my father from this time, Joanna writes: *Thank you so much for the flowers. It was a very kind gesture, as was the book. I was very close to my mother & it has been really hard. The flowers were a kindness I appreciated at such a difficult time.* She signs this with her customary ideogrammatic *J* and then below this, in block letters: *JOANNA.*

1992

Joanna sends me $1,000 when I run out of money during a "semester abroad" in England. Worried I won't come back otherwise, she invites my English boyfriend to visit us for a month in the summer. She takes us camping in Ohio and we visit the Serpent Mound. She chooses to sleep in the car, giving my boyfriend and me the tent.

On July 4, Joanna watches fireworks in the backyard of
her uncle Don's place in Laurel, Montana. Also this year,
she has an affair with a man she dated a decade earlier. He
is involved with mounting an exhibition of erotic drawings by John Lennon, and he has a girlfriend. Joanna
sends him a drawing of herself masturbating, in the style
of Lennon. *Thinking of you*, she writes inside the card. He
scolds her, telling her this was very inappropriate. "Do you
know how many guys would love to get that?" she asks
me, hotly indignant.

For the first and only time, Joanna flies across the Atlantic
Ocean, to visit me when I'm living in London for the year.
She sleeps on the floor in my room for two weeks and we
go out together, drinking lager and lime at my local pub.
A guy I think is cute tries to pick Joanna up, and when
she's in "the loo," he asks me if we're related. He doesn't
believe me when I say she's my mother. ("FUCK OFF!"
he replies.) Joanna pays for her and me to spend a weekend in Paris, where we stay at a B & B that I found in a
guidebook—which accurately described the floral décor
as very "Laura Ashley." In the morning we drink cup after
cup of café au lait before we head to the art museums. In
the Louvre, we race around in search of the Venus de
Milo and *Mona Lisa* before the museum closes. In
November, I return to the US and move back in with
Joanna for a couple of months, working at U-Save Auto
Rental for one of Joanna's old boyfriends, an ex-Marine.

In January, my father picks up me and my stuff at
Joanna's house and drives me to my new apartment in
Chicago. About a month later, the fellow Joanna had
been dating for more than a year, a thirty-year-old non-
smoker who liked Veruca Salt, breaks up with her. She
tells me, "The problem with dating younger guys is that
they always think of you as older."

1996	My appendix bursts shortly before my boyfriend and I are set to move in together. Joanna spends two weeks by my side, and I suspect my surgeon has a crush on her. "Why is she moving to Florida?" he asks me. "She shouldn't move to Florida. Florida is for old people." Joanna jokes that she lived with my boyfriend before I did; my boyfriend thinks this is an inappropriate joke. My mother moves to Boca Raton so that she can be close to her father and some of her extended family. The publishing company in Detroit where she has worked for seventeen years throws her a party and buys her a straw hat and two Pewabic Pottery tiles as mementos. She quickly finds a job in Florida, designing ads for a trade publisher specializing in magazines pitched at the produce industry. She piles up stock images of oranges, stock images of broccoli. She closes on a condo on December 20. For a month, she dates a guy from Long Island, and he buys her a VCR for Christmas. After I tell her I think he's annoying, she breaks up with him. He asks for the VCR back, which she thinks is fair. Though Joanna continues to attract male attention in her cropped T-shirts and tight white jeans, she never dates anyone again.
1997	Joanna and I spend a few days in Key West, floating up and down the beach, drinking cocktails. We pet Hemingway's six-toed cats, enjoy conch fritters and margaritas at Jimmy Buffett's Margaritaville, and watch the sunset with all the other tourists.
1998	In August, Joanna's father dies of leukemia in a hospital in Florida, several hours after she had gone home to get some sleep. On October 9, I send Joanna a card featuring a vintage French advertisement illustrated by Théophile A. Steinlen, much like one that hung in a frame in Joanna's various kitchens over the years. The illustration shows a young blond girl about to feed six excited cats a saucer of *crème*. I write: *I'm sorry that we've*

been fighting. I think that we are both going through hard times on our own right now, which we are bringing into our relationship. It makes me especially sad because it always upset Grandpa when we fought and I can clearly picture the look of displeasure on his face when he'd say, "Girls, stop it." Joanna will later store this card in a Ziploc bag, after covering the line *I'm so proud you are my mother* with two blank mailing labels and a strip of tape.

I send Joanna two postcards, after meeting Mike's family in Nova Scotia. On the back of a picture of Peggy's Cove, I write: *it's where they filmed much of that* Titanic *movie that made you cry.* In October, Joanna turns fifty and takes me to Disney World as a present to herself. We scream down Splash Mountain. Over Christmas, Mike and I visit her in Florida. We visit an amusement park where captive killer whales perform tricks for fish.

After I move to New York City in June, Joanna visits the city for the first time. While I'm at work, she goes to museums and takes a boat tour in which she takes many snapshots of the downtown skyline. I resentfully agree to go to the top of the Empire State Building with her, and she photographs me wearing the pair of Bulgari sunglasses I scored for free from work.

When Joanna hears the news that a plane has flown into the World Trade Center in New York, she calls me at work to make sure I'm okay. She visits as soon as it is possible to do so. A photograph she had taken of the Twin Towers from her sightseeing cruise appears in the magazine where she works.

While my mother is visiting me at the end of August, Mike and I decide to move to Toronto in September. "So this is my last trip to New York," she says sadly. Before the year is over, she visits me in Canada while Mike is on tour

1999

2000

2001

2002

and discloses that her brother Allan abused her. It is the
first and only time she will talk about this with me.

2003
According to my journal, on March 20 I dream that my
mother and I are in a car on an empty highway when we
realize nuclear bombs are about to be dropped. I say, "I'm
sorry, it's too late now." I wonder if we will feel any pain.
Everything goes white and I say, "I love you, Mom," and
she says, "I love you, Damian," and then I wake up.

2004
On February 12, Joanna receives a certificate in recognition of achieving a first-degree black belt in tae kwon do.
I visit her for two days at the end of July; it's my first trip
to Florida in two years.

2005
Joanna attends my graduation for my MFA in poetry
and buys the programme director, my thesis adviser, a
beer to thank him for mentoring me. I'm a little nervous
about people meeting her. I worry people will say, "Oh,
now I get it."

2006
On September 19, Joanna sends me an email that reads
*I gave blood today and passed out very bad and I am not
hitting on all cylinders right now.* She is trying to sell her
house. She wants to move to upstate New York to be
closer to me. She feels as if the house will never sell. On
October 13 she writes: *Anyway while your thinking of a
job for me remember I have had 27.5 years of experience in
magazine work.* A few weeks later: *I'm sorry my brain is
going to the dogs.*

2007
Joanna gives me her mother's gold band when I tell her
that Mike and I are going to elope. As a wedding gift,
Joanna buys me a much-needed computer.

2008
Joanna is serious about writing a science fiction book
pitched at a young-adult readership. Her New Year's

resolutions: *I am going to be calmer this year and get enough sleep . . . I bought a Tai Chi tape for once a week or so for calming purposes. I am also going to do other things for calming purposes. Particularly the book you gave me. I have decided that within the year I will finish my book and the one illustration I decided to do for the cover. Then I will see what I can do about getting it published or making emotional adjustments to not being able to get it published. When it is done fail or fly I will be starting another one. I find it more fun than I thought it would be. Plus you don't fully fail until you really worked for some time really hard and have tried all ways. Failure is not failure anyway. Not doing is failing.*

Joanna's brother Allan dies at the age of seventy. In September, the surviving siblings meet in Detroit to bury his ashes over my grandfather's grave. Later, her sister will tell me how Joanna broke down and sobbed. Later, Joanna will say, "When he died, I did not shed a tear."

In October, one of Joanna's co-workers calls to tell me she is worried because Joanna is making big mistakes on tasks she has completed skilfully for thirteen years. "Will you call her and see if she's okay?" she asks me. I reach out, but Joanna insists she is fine. I'm not sure what to do. She visits at Christmas and, in a moment of frustration with me, pulls a blanket over her head.

2009

Joanna sells her house in Florida and moves to upstate New York, buying a house in a suburb not far from Niagara Falls, close to the Canadian border. At the end of the year, she loses her job and is diagnosed with moderate dementia.

2010

Joanna lives for months at a time with different relatives until moving into an assisted-living facility at the end of the year. Two of her three cats die, and I place the third, named Marisol, with a writer in Toronto.

2011

2012	Joanna hides all of her money in her closet. Not long after her birthday, she becomes a grandmother.
2013	Joanna barricades the door to her room with a table, then a chair, then stacks of boxes.
2014	I work with a lawyer to try to keep my mother from getting pushed out of the assisted-living facility and into an under-resourced nursing home. In the notes from a psychiatric evaluation on February 7: *Episodes of paranoia and agitation and delusion-driven behavior. She notes she sleeps good. No death wishes.*
2015	Joanna moves into an under-resourced nursing home and refuses, for a time, to let anyone wash her.
2016	Marisol the artist dies. Joanna no longer knows or cares who this is.
2017	After twenty months and countless rejections from every nursing home I can find, Joanna is finally accepted into a nice facility on Midsummer's Day. Months later, she lands in the hospital after a twenty-minute seizure. Her speech never completely returns.
2018	Joanna and I sit together in the quiet corner of the locked unit at her nursing home, singing along to James Taylor: "I feel fine anytime she's around me now . . . She's around me now . . . all the time . . . And when I'm well you can tell . . . she's been with me now . . . She's been with me now . . . a long long time."
2019	Though her ability to communicate through language is almost gone, when I tell her I love her at the end of a visit, she replies clearly, "I love you too, sweetheart." She turns seventy in October.

```
XXXXXX                                        XXXXXX
 XXXXXX                                      XXXXXX
  XXXXXX                                    XXXXXX
   XXXXXX                                  XXXXXX
    XXXXXX                                XXXXXX
     XXXXXX                              XXXXXX
      XXXXXX                            XXXXXX
       XXXXXX                          XXXXXX
        XXXXXX                    XXXXXX
         XXXXXX                 XXXXXX
          XXXXXX   XXXXXX
           XXXXXXXXXX
          XXXXXX   XXXXXX
         XXXXXX                 XXXXXX
        XXXXXX                    XXXXXX
       XXXXXX                          XXXXXX
      XXXXXX                            XXXXXX
     XXXXXX                              XXXXXX
    XXXXXX                                XXXXXX
   XXXXXX                                  XXXXXX
  XXXXXX                                    XXXXXX
 XXXXXX                                      XXXXXX
XXXXXX                                        XXXXXX
```

HOW MUCH OF my mother's story was ever within my reach?

X is the sign that denies entry. X is the sinkhole in every unsolved formula. X is the shape of the eyes when cartoon characters die, their diaphanous souls drifting upwards, harps in their hands. X is the puckered portal to oblivion itself. X is the censor's black mark through disappeared data. X stands for all the things I will never, can never, know about my mother and my relationship with her, the exact lines of where she ends and I begin.

Every version of the story I try to follow to its conclusion splinters into a crossroads. Which way did she go? What kind of girl was she? What kind of woman? All my questions lead back to X.

I don't know all of "the gory details"—as my father called them—of the abuse my mother suffered as a child at the hands of her brother, or what further acts of violence may have passed between her and other men in her life. I'll never know what role, if any, a head injury may have had in the development of her frontal-temporal dementia. I don't know if I'll get the disease myself—and if I do get it, how old I might be when I begin my slide into the dark. I don't know, for that matter, that the disease hasn't already started its slow transformation of my brain. ("It's a twenty-year disease," one of my cousins said cheerfully.) There's no way to know what will happen. There is, however, one fact I do know: I carry a copy of the ApoE4 gene.

This doesn't mean that I'm doomed. It does mean I'm more likely to be doomed, that I have a higher risk of developing dementia by the time I reach the age of eighty-five than someone who doesn't carry a copy of this gene. But there are people who carry the gene who never end up with dementia, and there are people with dementia who don't carry the gene. So what does this information, which I received after taking a test I ordered over the Internet, really give me? Well, for one, it gives me an incentive to work harder at all the lifestyle choices believed to lower one's risk: I drink tea, I exercise, I meditate, I eat greens and sweet potatoes and blueberries. I spend a lot of money at the health food store on supplements: I take capsules of the medicinal mushroom lion's mane, high-dosage turmeric, something called bacopa and the most expensive fish oil available, which my naturopath assures me contains the least amount of contaminants.

My mother, too, took fish-oil capsules. She, too, ate well and exercised: she earned a martial arts black belt in her fifties; she forced her brother Roger and his wife to go on long, brisk walks every night after dinner. She completed at least one different crossword puzzle every day for ten years.

After I had taken the genetic test, I decided to buy a kit for my mother too, to see if she carried one or two copies of the ApoE4 gene. I hoped to find out that she carried two copies, that her risk factor was measurably, demonstrably, higher than mine. I visited her in Buffalo, bringing with me the plastic tube the genetic-test company had sent. I tried to explain to my mother what I wanted her to do. "Just spit in it," I told her, as I mimed spitting into my hand. She looked at me, brought the tube to her mouth and tentatively blew on it, the way you would blow across the top of a glass of water in order to produce a musical note.

One night back home, when Mike was away on tour and I was snuggling with Levi as he fell asleep, Levi said, "I don't ever want to leave you. I will have a lot of money when I get older so that if you ever have to go into the hospital, I can go with you. If you lose your memory, like Grandma Jo-Jo," he said, adding firmly, "but I don't think you will."

"That's sweet," Mike told me in the morning, after I relayed this story over the phone. "Now I want to hear more about this money he's going to have."

❦

EVER SINCE JOANNA became sick, I have been afraid. I watch myself closely, tracking each forgetful moment and—in some ways this is worse—the creeping fog that frequently nests in my head. The fog wants me to go back to bed, to give up on writing. There are days when I believe I am finally entering the future I've always dreamed of for myself, for my family; but then I think, no. I wasted so much time chasing my own tail, and now whatever abilities I might have developed are fading more each day. My idea of what

I want out of this life, how I want to spend whatever time I might have, is taking on a red-hot glow of urgency. As I'm writing this book, I can't help but wonder, am I fooling myself? Like my mother, who typed and typed her young-adult novel into an out-of-date graphic design application on her computer. When I tried to convert the text for her book into Word, so I could print it out for her, the file became corrupted. I sat at my desk and scrolled through hundreds of pages of random, meaningless symbols. In typography, this stream of unreadable marks is called dingbats.

I'm still learning to draw the line between my mother's life and my own.

"I wish I didn't find everything so frightening," Joanna said to me out of the blue one day, her voice even as a still pond. It was one of the last clear sentences I heard her utter. The idea of facing the same erasure, of slowly losing my memories, my language, my connections—what the fox taught the Little Prince to call "ties"—frightens me too. I am tied to Mike, I am tied to Levi, I am tied to my mother. The vision of my mind filling with long strings of Xs scares me more than the thought of death.

If I can make it to my eighties. If I can make it until Levi is grown up and has established himself. If.

We never know how much time. We always want more.

I have a friend whose father was diagnosed with the early stages of dementia in his late seventies. She doesn't want to know if she carries the gene. She is a firm believer that genetics are not predestination. When I found out the results of my genetic test, we texted back and forth. At the same time, we typed: *Of course, you can always end up getting hit by a bus.* And also: *(Why is it always a bus? Haha).*

Haha.

FROM THE TIME he was an infant in my arms, I have read Levi all of my mother's favourite stories: *Alice in Wonderland, The Wind in the Willows, Winnie-the-Pooh*, all seven books in the Harry Potter series. We are now reading Tolkien's Lord of the Rings trilogy. My father gave me his boxed paperback set when I saw him a few years ago, and I found one of my mother's drawings in it. Six lines of a song from the book beside a tall, leafy birch tree, her initial *J* hovering above blades of soft grass.

We watch the screen adaptions of these stories too. I don't like the Disneyfication of *Winnie-the-Pooh* in the cartoons; for me, all of the characters' features look rounder, exaggerated, in these versions. I find the illustrations in the original books more alive, more delicate in expression, more evocative of the vulnerable smudge between real and not-real. But even in this diluted form, Winnie-the-Pooh's sweet self-castigation strikes my heart, as he struggles to remember something, knocking himself on his stuffed head. "Think! Think! Think!"

These days, a chill runs through me every time I mix up words. For a while, I kept a record of every slip. I couldn't remember the word *gateway*. I said *salsa* when I meant *hummus*. I said *rescinded* instead of *redundant*.

I became so concerned that I made an appointment for a full cognitive health evaluation. There was an interview, a paper test. I had to draw the hands on a clock, I had to count backwards from one hundred by seven, and then I was asked to repeat back strings of numbers. It was stressful. I didn't feel as if I was performing well at all. Toward the end of the exam, the doctor said,

"I want you to name as many animals as you can before I say stop." I burst out laughing.

One day I was home alone with Levi, following five different complicated health food recipes in the kitchen while Levi played in the living room. I was melting a quarter cup of coconut oil on the stove for a high-fibre, grain-free seed loaf when Levi called me and I went to him. He asked me to read to him from his dinosaur book, and I totally spaced out about the oil on the stove—until the smoke alarm went off. When I ran back into the kitchen, there was a column of flame three feet high rising out of the saucepan. I panicked. Wait, how do you put out a grease fire? I know, not water, not water. Levi was screaming, "Make it stop, Mama, make it stop!" At a loss, I threw a glass of water at it from the kitchen doorway—the flames shot up in the air and then went out. A small black mark on the ceiling.

Later, I texted Mike, *I'm really worried about my brain.* He texted back, *Dude no offense, but you've been burning pots since I met you.*

habit / habitation / habituation / hack
hackle / hair / half / hallelujah / Halloween
hallucination / hallways / hammock
handwriting / happiness / harassment
harbinger / harmony / haunt / haze / headaches
headlights / health / heartbreak / heat / heaven
hedge / heirloom / help / helplessness / hemlock
hemorrhage / herb / heritability / hermeticism
heron / hesitation / hex / hider / highjacker
highroad / highway / him / hinderance / history
hobbit / hold / hole / hollyhock / H O M E
homecoming / honesty / honey / honeypot
honour / hook / hope / horizon / horn / horoscope
horror / horses / hospital / hospitality / host
hostage / hound / householder / hue / hug
humiliation / hummingbird / hunt / hurricane
hurt / hustle / hygiene / hyperbole
hypersensitivity / hypnotism / hypocrisy / hysteria

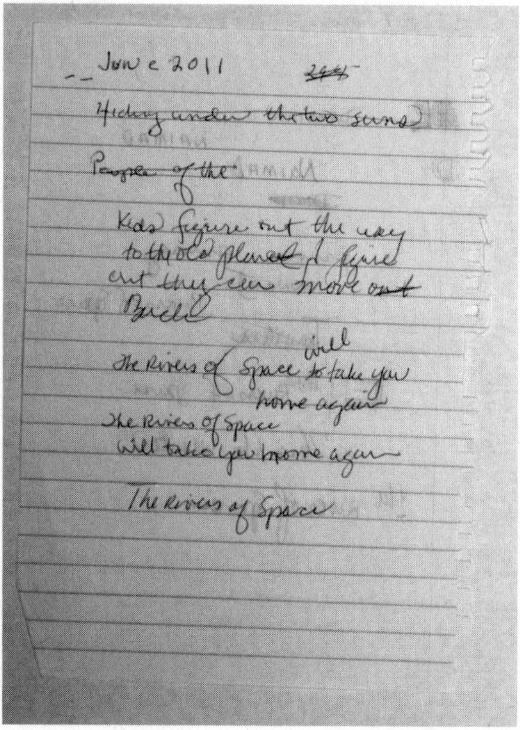

JOANNA'S NOTEBOOK, 2010

The rivers of space will take you home again
The rivers of space will take you home again
The rivers of space

"YOU KNOW, MAMA, there are things worse than death in the muggle world too. That's a real thing," Levi tells me.

We are playing a Harry Potter game as I fold the laundry. In the game, I am folding clothes and towels at Hogwarts. I am helping out the house elves. I think of what my mother would have given to be able to play Harry Potter games with Levi.

"Oh," I said. "That's interesting. Like what, do you think?"

"Like Grandma Jo-Jo's disease. The forgetting disease is badder than death," he said evenly.

I stopped folding the shirt in my hand and looked at my son. He was sitting on the bed, watching me work.

"Because she can't remember?" I asked, my throat tight.

"It's not just that she can't remember things. Grandma Jo-Jo can't—" He paused, searching for the right words.

"*Do* things," he finished, with an emphasis that bordered on exasperation.

"I know it's hard that you can't play with Grandma Jo-Jo," I said to him.

"I can play with Grandma Jo-Jo," he corrected me. "I just have to play with her in a different way."

❧

AUTHOR AND COMIC book artist Lynda Barry asks, "Why is there anxiety about a past we cannot change? The top of the mind has no answer for this."

A year ago in the fall, I travelled to Montana, to see the place where my mother was born and visit my cousins there. When I spoke with Mike and Levi one night, Levi cried out from the bathtub over the speakerphone, "Your kitty-cat is going down the drain! Help me!"

Levi loved pretending to be a cat. I called back to him, "I've got you! I'm pulling you up to safety!"

"You're just on the phone," he reminded me.

There was a moment of silence.

"It's too late! Your kitty-cat went down the drain!"

"Oh honey—"

"Come home right now!" he yelled at the phone. "Tonight!"

❧

IN MONTANA, I felt closer to death.

I drove alone every day through long stretches of dead grass and sagebrush, through canyons and rimrock, past tabletop mountains and peaks named Bear Tooth and Crazy. I made lists of the animals I saw along the roads: horses and cows, of course, and many deer, a fox, a bald eagle. I felt it would be easy to accidentally die here, on these roads. It wasn't just the possibility of a devastating crash, it was the shape of the space around me: cold, and hard. Unforgiving, I thought. Unyielding. How did people survive before the soft comforts of well-insulated, heated homes, heated cars? Only through relationships.

My cousin Rachel and I visited the old cemetery where our great-grandmother Ivy was buried. This great-grandmother's older sister, Bessie, had died of diphtheria at five years of age, in that first winter on the homestead. The family was living in a tarpaper shack, and Bessie's body had to be buried on the land until a cemetery was established the following year. The headstone, a small, elegant obelisk, reads *Born Oct. 19, 1893. Died Feb. 9, 1899. Tread softly by / the grave of One / our hearts had / learned to love.* The day my cousin and I visited the gravesite, it was so cold that my right hand became chapped in the short time we stood there and didn't heal until I had returned home to Toronto.

To get to Rachel's house, which was relatively close to where I was staying, took me about twenty-five minutes. I loved my solitary drives, and I also couldn't wait for them to end. I wanted to soak up and store as much of the landscape's energy as I could, and then hurry home, back to Toronto, where death is buried under the density of human activity, under emails and coffee dates, under school drop-offs, laundry and paperwork, and the daily problem of dinner.

Driving around Montana, I crossed the Yellowstone River and made several pilgrimages to the area around my great-great-grandfather's homestead on Rock Creek. I'd brought a photograph of Rock Creek with me, one I'd kept from my mother's collection. On the back, someone had written: "Where Allan and I crossed on horseback."

❧

AMONGST HER SIBLINGS, my mother had the distinction of being the only one born in Montana. But it was her second brother, Roger, eight years her senior, who eventually wrote about that time. He typed up all of his memories of the summer the family lived in the Little House on Rock Creek, and illustrated these stories with family photos, some of which I'd never seen before Rachel let me borrow her copy. Roger had bound and sent it to her while in the early stages of Alzheimer's.

My great-grandmother Ivy's father had built the Little House after his wife died. It was tiny at first—only two small rooms. My own grandmother had called it the Doll House. And though my mother had been too young to remember the time she and her family had spent there, Montana still loomed large in her private mythology. She visited Montana twice as a child, during the 1950s, and once again as an adult in the 1990s. She felt it was significant to have been born there. Among her many semi-precious rocks and crystals, she always had a prized piece or two of "Montana agate."

When she was in her mid-forties, my mother wrote a young-adult mystery about a fourteen-year-old girl from Michigan named Devin who goes to live with her grandmother in Montana for a summer and gets caught up in the task of solving a murder. The character of Devin was based on me, and the character of the murderer was based on a man with whom Joanna had had an ill-fated affair. Years later she decided the story was no good and threw it out. I still remember a scene where an older teenaged boy—not the murderer, we learn later—follows Devin to a desolate place, rolling a penny at her from the deep shadows, where he remains hidden, just to spook her. She runs off and he laughs as he watches her. I wish I could read it again; I wonder what I'd think of it now.

Ivy, Joanna's grandmother, had been born in Montana in 1896. In 1981, Ivy's obituary ran locally with the headline FIRST WHITE GIRL BORN IN THE JUDITH BASIN. During my time in Montana, I thought often about Ivy, and I would whisper to myself, "My mother's mother's mother." Perhaps I hoped that, by returning to the location of my mother's birth, I might reconnect to the place where the line of mothers pointed back.

❦

MY MOTHER'S COUSIN—Rachel's father, Fred—suggested we have a meal together while I was in town. We decided on lunch, so I could be off the roads by the time the sun set, and we found a restaurant where I could order something in line with the dementia-prevention diet I had copied out of a book. I sat beside Cousin Fred and we spoke intensely about family. I quizzed him about various details of Ivy's biography, and his impressions of my mother.

"I'm afraid I don't remember your mother well at all," he told me. And he had no memory of the trip my mother had made to Montana in the 1990s, after I'd moved to Chicago.

"That's strange," I said. "I have this photo at home of my mother with her sister, and I was sure Uncle Roger had taken it in Montana sometime around then."

Fred shook his head. He told me how my grandfather, his uncle, had been a gentle and affectionate man, and a great storyteller. His aunt Jeanne—my grandmother—had been the one who'd introduced him to my mother when they were children. "She put her arm around me and said, 'Now I know Joanna is a bit younger than you, but you should get to know her. I think you'll find her very interesting.'

"I got the feeling that your mother was very special to everyone," Fred said. As we chatted, he sketched a map of the homestead on the paper tablecloth in front of us. Before we left, I carefully tore it off, and took it with me.

"Have you seen the home movies?" he asked as he settled the bill, his treat. "They were transferred to video and I have a copy of them at home. I can also go through and pull out any old photos I might have of your mom."

We made plans for me to drop by his house the next day.

❦

"I'M AFRAID I lied to you!" Fred said with a smile when I arrived at his door. After our meal, he'd gone home and pulled up a video his father had made on the Fourth of July in 1993—and there was Joanna. He pushed the tape into the square mouth of his VHS player.

The footage buzzed with the grainy decay of video, but there she was indeed—my mother in her mid-forties, the same age I was as I watched. Wearing a striped shirt and small gold hoop earrings, she smiled, exuding a low-hum nervous energy, her eyes darting down or away whenever she noticed the camera. She was still wearing her hair well past her shoulders, with full bangs across her forehead. She seemed the most herself, the most natural and unselfconscious, when she was cuddling someone's new kitten in her arms. The resemblance between her and me was undeniable.

"I have to admit, at first I thought that might actually be you," Fred told me. "And then I heard someone ask her if she had a picture of you, and I figured it out."

He also played me a video cassette my grandfather had distributed amongst the family in the late eighties, when the old home movies he had shot throughout the 1950s had been converted from Super 8. My mother was a toddler, then four years old, then six years old. My grandmother had dressed Joanna in ruffled shirts and dresses. In almost every shot my mother was wearing pink, frothy, frilly things. This surprised me. As an adult, my mother's femininity was always understated. She was most comfortable in tight jeans and a fitted shirt, a little black dress for a date. And she had dressed me in overalls and corduroy newsboy hats when I was little. I had never seen her like this. I had never seen her wear pink. I had never seen her so girly.

On the television screen, she performed for the camera happily in every scene, grinning and dancing and scampering about. There was footage of the family camping, footage of them in Montana. Footage of all four kids assembling on the lawn in front of the house in Michigan that I grew up in too. Allan was probably not yet out of the house; perhaps these movies were taken just before he joined the navy. As they arranged themselves into formation for a photo, my mother ran straight to Allan and then turned to stand in front of him. She was six years old. Allan's hands rose up to hold her in place by the shoulders. They were both smiling.

After the movies were finished, Fred and I sat in the kitchen and looked through meticulously labelled files of black-and-white photographs. I skimmed through the ones with my mother and grandmother, setting aside those I'd like to have scanned. "Honestly, that woman always looked like she was going to the opera," Fred said, with a good-natured laugh, about my grandmother, Aunt Jeanne to him. He clearly preferred the more down-to-earth style of his mother, my grandmother's younger sister, who'd spent more time out west due to her asthma.

As I looked through a file marked "Ivy," a very old photo that was cracked down the middle caught my attention. It showed a tough-looking woman in a high-necked, dark dress with puffed sleeves. On the back was the caption "my mother's mother" in Ivy's handwriting.

"This is a photograph of Ivy's mother's mother?" I asked Fred.

"Yes," he said.

"That's so strange she wrote it this way. I've been thinking about her as my 'mother's mother's mother' on this whole trip," I told him. "So, this is a photograph of my great-great-great-grandmother?"

"Yes," he said.

"That means this is a picture of my mother's mother's mother's mother's mother," I said, stunned. My mind spun, imagining the direct link, body to body. Mothers all the way back.

Ivy's mother was Eva. No one left in our family knows what Eva's mother's name was. I'm guessing that Ivy herself had never known this woman, as she hadn't written her name, or even "my grandmother," on the back of the photograph. This woman was a ghost to Ivy, just as Ivy is a ghost to me.

Ghosts all the way back.

❦

ON THE PLANE home, I held a suede-bound copy of the *Collected Verse of Rudyard Kipling*. Cousin Fred had discovered that I was a poet and pressed it into my hands, making me promise that I would pass this volume down to Levi, that I would keep it in the family. It had been Ivy's, and on a thin strip of paper still tucked inside she had written, "This is one of my priceless treasures."

I am still finding these kinds of notes in my own books. At home in my office, I pull down a copy of a book called *Poetry Speaks*, a large anthology that came with audio CDs of poets reading their work. My mother had bought it for me for my thirtieth birthday, when I still lived in New York. A pale, pebble-textured piece of pink paper was folded inside with my mother's handwriting on it.

I am totally swamped or I'd write something wonderful

Then a long, squiggly arrow pointed off the page—a cue for me to flip the paper over for more.

Trust that I love you and that I am always here for you and always have been. I can't believe you're 30— How did that happen? Yesterday—you were a toddler figuring out the locks on the drawers in the kitchen. If you can figure out how to be happy regardless of what life hits you with you will have succeeded. You have already exceeded my dreams for you and of you.

Love,
Mama

❦

I COOK DINNER for Levi and myself, chopping red onion and kale, frying them in coconut oil in a heavy, black cast iron pan. The purple of the onion, the green of the kale. I wash the dishes, wipe down the counter. The late afternoon sun glows through the small pane of orange-stained glass with a picture of blooming marjoram on it that hangs from the same brown velvet ribbon from which it once hung in the window over the sink in my grandmother's kitchen.

Levi and I pick rose and calendula petals from the garden in the backyard. The calendula petals like tender needles of light glow in the bowl.

The more alive I feel, the less afraid I am of dying.

"Is it morning time?" Levi asks me.

"No, it's afternoon. Do you want me to teach you how to tell time, honey?" I ask him.

"Do not. Never ever teach me time. I don't want to know time."

Since Levi was three years old, he and I have collaborated on little books together. I write down things he says while he draws. I find that if I'm lazy and wait until after he finishes the drawing, what he'll tell me about it is much less interesting than his real-time commentary. Like a poem, the drawing is an event. The drawing is alive to him in the moments that he chooses each next direction. So we collaborate, side by side. I work to catch what he's thinking as he makes each decision. "Kitty-cats are falling from the sky!" he'll say, as he draws dark balls in streaking formation. We make an abecedarian book that he calls *ABC CATS. A* is for American Shorthair. *B* is for Bengal. "*S* has to be Siamese," he told me. "For Ivan."

Ivan. I've taught him the name of my grandparents' last cat.

I make a story of my life as a mother. The story makes me.

After dinner, but before bedtime, Levi looks through the photos on my phone.

"Mama, let's say we take pictures of everything we love," he says.

His hair is long, and the tips of the curls have bleached coppery gold from the summer sun. "He really looks like your mother," Mike has told me many times. Our son's large, round, dark eyes, something about the shape of his chin.

Yes, I think. Let's take pictures of everything we love. Like me, Levi wants to take pictures, to document, to remember. He wants to hold everything. He doesn't want anything he loves to slip away. Yes, honey, I think, let's remember everything we love. Let's. But before I can agree, he finishes his thought—

"And let's say we love everything."

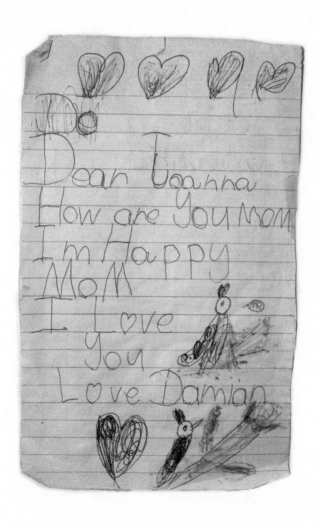

Dear Joanna
How are You Mom
I'm Happy
MoM
I Love
You
Love Damian

NOTE ON THE TEXT

THE LISTS OF words at the beginning of each chapter are made entirely of nouns. In cases where a word could be misread as a verb or adjective, imagine either the definite or indefinite article before it, such as "the missing" or "a muddle."

ACKNOWLEDGEMENTS

THANK YOU TO Joanna, who gave me everything. I promise not to forget.

Thank you to Michael and Levi, who always lead me home.

This project would have been impossible without Lynn Henry, who believed in it from the beginning and who continued to believe in it, and in me, even when I lost faith. Thank you for giving my book a beautiful home and for all you did to make it better. I am so grateful.

Thank you to Rick Meier, Kate Sinclair, John Sweet, Sue Sumeraj, Suzanne Brandreth, Stephen Myers, Anne Collins, Kristin Cochrane and all at Knopf Canada and Penguin Random House.

Thank you to Jess Atwood Gibson for your generosity and friendship, and for your brilliant and tireless attention to these pages in their many stages.

Thank you to Marilyn Biderman, Suzanne Buffam, Samantha Haywood, Mathew Henderson, Canisia Lubrin, Hoa Nguyen, Ansley Simpson, Leanne Betasamosake Simpson, Alex Tigchelaar, Nancy Salter and Margaux Williamson for encouragement, support, and wise counsel.

Thank you to all who offered me the space to work away from my wonderful family, including Madhur Anand, the Atwood-Gibsons, Amanda Burt, Kate Boothman, Judith Coombe, Gisele Gordon and Archer Pechawis, Greg Keelor, Kathryn Kuitenbrouwer, Kat Taylor-Small and Justin Small, Tova Smith and Evan Newman, Zoe Whittall and anyone else I've forgotten. I am also grateful for stays at the Banff Centre's Leighton Artist Colony, Artscape Gibraltar Point and the Al and Eurithe Purdy A-Frame. Thank you, thank you, thank you to Janet "Monster Pillow" Hoy for holding my kid while I tried to write.

Thank you to my father.

Thank you to the rest of my family—through blood and through love. Special thanks to my Montana cousins, Rachel, Sharon, Jody, and Fred, who welcomed me so completely.

Thank you to all of the professionals and volunteers who have helped care for my mother and to all of the professionals and volunteers around the world who care for people with dementia.

I am grateful for the fact that this book was assisted by grants from the Canada Council of the Arts, the Ontario Arts Council and the Toronto Arts Council.

Some material from this book appeared in a short presentation I gave as part of The Walrus Talks Better Living event in Toronto on October 29, 2019. This talk was subsequently published in *The Walrus*. A version of the poem "Thursday, A Grand Total" appeared in *Canadian Art* magazine and "Songs to Sing to an Estranged Lover While Secretly Pregnant" appeared on *The Puritan*. Thank you to the respective editors.

Please note that "Blue Bayou," which I refer to in the text as a Linda Ronstadt song, was written by Roy Orbison and Joe Melson. The sheet music my mother used to learn to play guitar had a photo of Linda Ronstadt on it, which explains my childhood confusion.

DAMIAN ROGERS is the author of two acclaimed books of poetry: *Dear Leader* (2015), which was named one of the best books of 2015 by the CBC and the *Globe and Mail*, and was a finalist for the Ontario Trillium Poetry Prize; and *Paper Radio* (2009), which was shortlisted for the Pat Lowther Memorial Prize. She holds a graduate degree from the Bennington Writing Seminars in Bennington, Vermont, and has published work in many magazines and online journals, including *Boston Review*, *Brick*, *The Walrus*, *Hazlitt*, *White Wall Review*, *Event*, *Four Way Review*, *Taddle Creek*, *Riddle Fence*, *Toronto Star*, *Maisonneuve*, *Salt Hill* and more. Damian teaches creative writing at Ryerson University. She lives in Toronto.

1. American BlackBear 2. ALASKAN BROWN Bear
3. Kodiak Bear 4. SLOTH Bear 5. Specticaled
. Bear
6. Polar Bear 7. Sun Bear 8. Grizzley Bear
~~9. Polar Bear 10. 5 Polar Bear 10.~~
9. welsh terrier 10. welsh Springer spaniel
11. Jack Russel 12. ~~te~~ Akita
13. Blood Hound 14. ALASKAN MALAMUTE
15. Yorkshire terrier 16. German ~~Steper~~
She pard
17. Siamese Cat 18. Burmese Cat
19. ~~Abysinian~~ Abysinian cat
20. Main coon cat 21. Eyptian Maw
Cat
22. Don Sphynx ~~cat~~ - Hairless.
23. Bombay cat - (BLACK) ~~24.~~
24. Manx Cat - Short tail - Apeared Naturally
300 years
25. Kangaroo ~~Sta~~ small ago
26. Tree Kangaroo 27. Red Kangaroo
28. Golden Jackal 29. Black-Backed
Jackal
30. Side Stripe Jackals
31. American Buffalo 32. American
Bison
33. Snow Leopard 34. Clouded Leopard
35. Leopard Lynx 36. Arabian Horse
37. Arabian Camel 38. Bactraisn Camel
39. Wild Margay Cat 40. Wild Leopard Cat
41. Mule 42. Mole 43. Moose 44 Ostrige

45. Weasel 46. Giraffe 47. Pygmie Horse

48. Osolot, 49. Big Horned Sheep

50. Fennic Fox - Big Ears /Keeps cool

51. Badger 52. Spotted Hyena 53. Gelata Baboon

54. Giant Panda Bear

55. Gray Mouse Lemur 56. Ringtail Lemur

57. Bob Cat 58. Black ~~Rhinasour~~ Rhinoceros

59. Rhino ~~Steel~~ white Rhinoceros

60. ~~Hippopo~~ Hippopotamus

61. Howeler Monkey 62. Mandrill Monkey

63. Artic Hare 64. Artic Fox 65. Artic (Ground Squirrel

66. Artic Musk-Oxen

67. Black Panther 68. Chimpanze

69 Jack Rabbit 70. Fennic Fox

71. Mountain Zebra ~~72. Giant Elephant Big Horned Sheep 5~~

73. Baird's Taper 74. Pigs/Swine

75. Armadillo 76. Jersey Cows

77. Asian Giraffe 78. Giant River Otters

79. Gibbon 80. Deer 81. Pussum

83. ~~Deer~~ 84. African Pgmie Hedge Hog

85. Gazelle 86. Porcupine

86. Puma 87. Lama 88 Lamb

72. Giant Elephant Shrew